THE LONG MOMENT

Giving A Voice to the Alzheimer's Mind:
A Caregiver's Guide

Richard Fenker, PhD

First Printing
July 2013

Cimarron International LLC
Cimarron Press
Copyright © 2013 Richard Fenker
All Rights Reserved

ISBN: 978-0-9894600-0-2

For Katherine, Emilou, and the Fenkers

To Dad, kind parent, loving friend, and generous being, who inspired this book

Preface

This book is written, in part, for the many thousands of Alzheimer's caregivers who offer time, love, and attention to their family members, friends, and partners with this insidious disease. I recognize, as most caregivers recognize, that this process, which may last a decade, is filled with uncertainty, frustration, and disappointment as you watch a normal, healthy mind and familiar personality decay into one controlled by the disease.

It is also written for the individual with the disease. What I am attempting to do with this book is to give a voice to the person suffering from Alzheimer's by describing how the disease corrupts the everyday process of living and sharing the same reality, but, at the same time, reminding you, the caregiver, how much of your partner is "still there" when the glass is viewed as half full rather than half empty.

The concept of a "long moment" is tied to the present tense rather than the past or the future. When you are living in the present with your partner, not trying to help them remember or recover a past that no longer exists, thousands of long moments are available to you. When you understand that your shared reality depends on different rules now and are willing to relinquish the demands that a verbal, logical, left-brain world places on Alzheimer's patients, you move a big step toward their world. When you are willing to stop evaluating and simply be present in the now, flowing with their needs, it transforms the dynamic of your relationship from me-you to "us" and replaces frustration with focused listening and unconditional kindness. Finally, when you are willing to acknowledge that this former friend or partner is now a stranger, but one you can love, comfort, and assist by building a new relationship, you have provided a most precious gift.

I am not an Alzheimer's expert but rather just an individual whose life has been impacted by family members dealing with Alzheimer's disease and also a scientist interested in human consciousness and how it operates under many conditions. We often think of consciousness as the one-dimensional, logical, conversational parts of our mind that are with us from waking in the morning to bedtime, yet this is absolutely not the case. Consciousness is complex and multidimensional and embraces all aspects of our physical and mental beings. At every moment in time, each of us has choices to make about our world, whether we are happy or unhappy, encouraged or discouraged, engaged or simply coasting along. Alzheimer's brings with it so much fear, uncertainty, and a fatalistic view (yes, it is true, they really are not going to recover) that it can short-circuit this normal process of choosing the best options and then acting accordingly.

My view is that a process that orients you in the direction of the most favorable, helpful, and loving outcomes is always available to you when you are ready, and by embracing it, you bring the blessing of many long moments to you and your partner and the gift of peace, despite the many difficulties you will face, to yourself.

Warm wishes to you as you provide the gifts of kindness, patience, and caring for your friend or partner with Alzheimer's disease, and also remember to offer the same blessings to yourself.

Richard Fenker

April 22, 2013

Contents

I Cannot Remember What I Forgot

I awakened this morning with a clear head,
Had a very fine breakfast,
And then made my plans for the day.
Oh my. What day is this?
I cannot remember what I forgot.

I enjoyed the trips we took with Aunt Betty.
They were filled with so much fun.
We visited some most interesting places.
I am sure we did.
I cannot remember what I forgot.

I miss you so much.
My heart soars when you visit.
Your love has added so much joy to my life.
Why are you here today?
I cannot remember what I forgot.

My life has meaning and purpose.
Writing this poem is part of my destiny.
It tells my story now.
What was my story before?
I cannot remember what I forgot.

I remember so much and so little.
But this really doesn't matter because
My life has been filled with joyful moments.
And I know this poem is holding one.
I cannot remember what I forgot.

—Anonymous

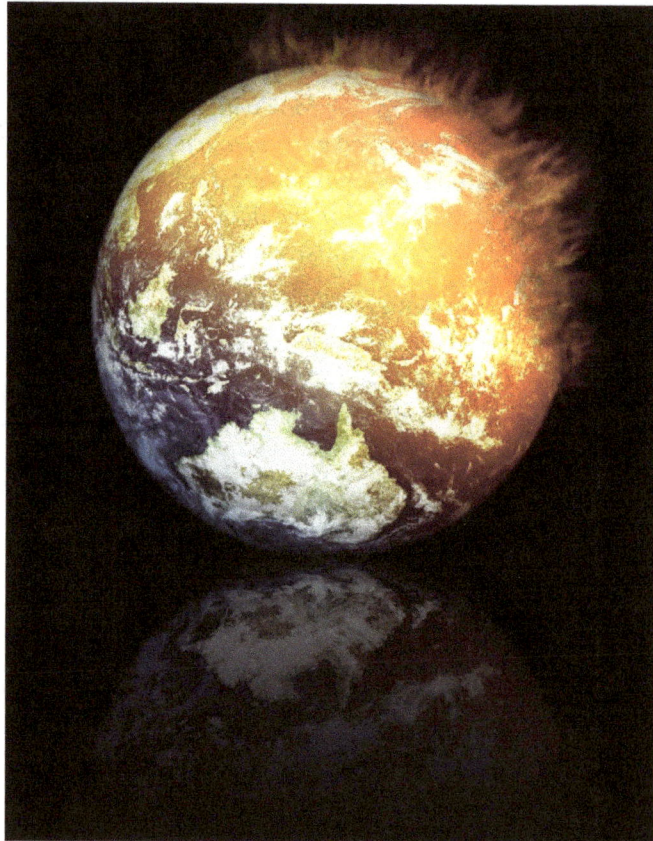

A Journey to the Planet Altzair

Introduction

My Story

The first time I can remember hearing the term *Alzheimer's disease* was in 1959 when my grandfather, Fodda, who had been struggling with dementia for some time, was finally given this diagnosis. It meant little more to me than my vague ideas around dementia, which meant largely forgetting things, missing names, and fuzzy cognitive skills—all associated with aging in my mind. So I heard this diagnosis, and unlike cancer or heart disease or stroke, it had no fear or anxiety associated with it. Fodda was aging. This was to be expected.

The next year I was away at college and the family gatherings at Grandmother's house were less and less frequent as was my opportunity to interact with Fodda. Then, in a letter from Mom, there is mention of Fodda being moved to a nearby nursing home because he needed more care than the family could provide. Nursing home, getting old, all of this seemed very normal to me. Soon I had graduated from college and was home for a month. Mom suggested that it was time I visited Fodda just so I would understand why he hadn't been in touch for so long.

The nursing home was an older building that had been converted into a hospital ward. It smelled of urine and sweat and old wood and moldy carpets, all of which contrasted with an undefined antiseptic scent that reminded me of a chemistry experiment gone amiss. And there was Fodda, ninety-three years old, sitting in a chair by his bed, looking healthy but unable to remember Mom or me and upset because we were strangers intruding in his space. I was shocked by the changes in him and by his inability to recognize who we were. Mom explained that this was a relatively good day. On bad days he refused to get out bed and was uncooperative with the staff and often belligerent. Fodda lived another two years. Occasionally he did recognize Mom and could communicate with her, but these skills diminished quickly. Dad was enormously frustrated with him. As his business partner, Dad had been dealing with the aging process for some years, frustrated by a legacy of business issues that could not be resolved.

When Fodda died, it was anti-climatic for me, as I was very seldom at home and thought of him as "gone" anyway, living in the nursing home and out of touch with my world. For Dad, however, it was a life-changing experience. He had watched as Fodda went from the beginnings of dementia to anxiety and frustration, as his capability to function and communicate diminished to the point of apathy and helplessness, leading eventually to the move to the nursing home. Every dimension of this was stressful for the family and no insurance at this time covered nursing home care.

Dad was concerned that he would follow in Fodda's footsteps and succumb to Alzheimer's disease as he aged, and he didn't want any part of this. He was open with this concern, and so soon after Fodda's death at ninety-five, we were all living with the fear of Alzheimer's, not so much for ourselves but for Dad. What it meant for me was that I was "tuned" to listen for any news related to Alzheimer's, such as friends or other individuals showing signs of the disease and the growing body of medical and scientific information about Alzheimer's disease and its impact on individuals and families.

Soon after Fodda's death, I took a teaching position as a professor at TCU with a special interest in nonverbal communication and human consciousness. What I had recognized personally and in teaching was how much information is shared in classroom interactions, personal relationships, individual and group counseling, sports, and many other activities outside of traditional, left-brain conversations (our normal communication process). Some fascinating research on classroom learning showed that students who had similar political beliefs and attitudes about life did much better in classes with professors who shared similar beliefs and that this effect was almost as strong a predictor as the students' previous academic performance.

At any moment in time our conscious and unconscious minds are processing much more information than we have an awareness of. Think of an iceberg. At least 90 percent of what is happening in the mind at any moment is below our level of awareness, especially when we are functioning in our traditional linear, conversational mode (which is most of the time). The idea that Alzheimer's disease was just another special case of this problem came from multiple sources, including Marshall McLuhan's work on media and how our choice of media shapes human consciousness as well as the growing body of knowledge on the evolution of human consciousness.

Although at the time it was a stray thought and didn't receive much attention, the idea popped into my mind that much of the fearfulness associated with Alzheimer's disease is analogous to the fear experienced by some people in meditation when everyday waking consciousness is temporarily suspended and they feel less in control. With this loss of control in the meditative state, some people relax and experience the joy and the peacefulness that comes from "letting go" while many others struggle as the talking mind insists on staying in charge. What Dad feared the most about Alzheimer's was the helplessness and *complete loss of control* coming at the end of a life built on working hard, saving, and investing in order to maintain control in the later years of life.

This idea was reinforced again a few years later in my work with public housing in urban settings and on reservations. What I learned over and over is that the primary issue is not crowding or some other social problem that we (society) project onto this situation, but rather it is the personal need for control by individuals and families in these settings. When a degree of control is present in the environment, even in very modest doses, people do OK. When it is not, they are frustrated.

The voice in me grew louder and louder. Mom and Dad were in their eighties now, and both, fortunately, remained mentally alert and showed no signs of Alzheimer's disease. However, many of their friends and family and my friends were not so lucky. The father of my partner for two years, Carol, was diagnosed with early Alzheimer's. Dad's sister, my aunt Emilou, who was close to us, moved to Florida with her daughter, Katherine, and soon was experiencing the early stage problems of memory loss and difficulty with everyday tasks such as dressing or preparing meals. Now at one hundred, Aunt Emilou, like her father, is physically healthy in many respects but suffering from the debilitating consequences of late stage Alzheimer's. Every time I visited Dad (which was weekly) in my mind was his fear of Alzheimer's. On each visit I was checking and thinking "Is he just a little dingy today or is this something more serious?"

One day, in 2000, just after both Mom and Dad had died, I was sitting quietly on the back porch of my mountain home in Fort Davis thinking about Dad and his last night with me. We spent hours together that last night, just talking about things in his life that we had shared, and as I held his hand, as he died, I thought how grateful I was for this last time together in a world that was filled with common memories and experiences.

Reflecting on the night my father passed on, a voice in my mind said to me, "You need to write a book on Alzheimer's disease. So much of the disease for both the person and the caregivers is about fear. The path to help them is to understand the role of consciousness here. That's the key to communication, which is the key to relinquishing the fear. You can help."

That was the genesis of this book.

The Ideal Minute: A Few Observations about Time

For twenty years in my TCU class States of Consciousness I used an exercise called "Ideal Time" with the students. Their assignment the first week was to plan and then experience whatever they would define as an "Ideal Minute" during the next week and then write a brief one-paragraph report on this episode. No one experienced any difficulty with this first task, and as you might expect, I received an array of reports about many pleasurable activities, long kisses, smoking a joint, eating ice cream, and hundreds of others.

In the second week the task was to plan and experience an "Ideal Hour" during the week. Once again, this presented little problem and most students loved the idea of planning and doing something that was deliberately enjoyable as part of an assignment. Many students chose activities at home that were missed because of busy schedules such as watching a favorite TV show, playing a sport, an activity with a friend, or, in many cases, intentionally resting or relaxing for an hour. Again, the feedback was very positive, but it was still not obvious to the students where this exercise was headed.

You may have already guessed the third week's exercise, which was to plan and experience an "Ideal Day." It was also at this point that the process began to break down for many students. My most dedicated students would plan a Saturday or Sunday activity such as a short trip, a picnic, a long date, and think it was practical to take the entire day for a pleasurable set of experiences. My adult classes were better here at scheduling all-day events but not by much. Reports this week often communicated the frustration of wanting to do the assignment but quickly recognizing that it was not realistic, at least with their current interpretation of "ideal."

By the time I gave the final assignment, to plan and experience an "Ideal Week" and report on the results, the point of the exercise was obvious to most students. If ideal time is based solely on pleasure and finding enjoyable activities to fill it, then the opportunities for living an ideal day were challeng-

4

ing, and to live an ideal week, impossible! Now, with this background, I was able to introduce the notion that ideal time is really about how you experience all moments in time, pleasurable or not, and that it is your reaction to these moments, not how much you enjoy them in a literal sense, that matters. If you go through life defining ideal time strictly in terms of pleasure or enjoyment, there is likely to be lots of "down time," which is not ideal. On the other hand, if you define time in a manner that is anchored to the moment and your reactions to that moment, virtually all time can be "ideal" and experienced as happy, enjoyable, and fulfilling. Dining, spending time with a partner, working, cleaning, or any other activity can be experienced as enjoyable if you choose to interpret it in that manner.

To illustrate this point, consider the problem of driving on busy city streets during rush hour. Is this an example of ideal time? Hardly, but with a simple twist in thinking about this experience you can turn the haste and frustrations of rush hour into just another experience. Normally when you are driving in traffic it is because you are going somewhere—home after work, shopping, to exercise, to pick up your children—and because your focus is on "getting there on time" everything that slows you down is interfering with this goal and therefore a source of stress or hassle. Try this simple exercise. Anytime you can for the next couple of weeks look for opportunities to drive in rush hour traffic. If you need to drive somewhere for a specific goal (such as driving home from work), give yourself an extra twenty minutes so time is not a problem, or, even better, find times when you can just be in the traffic with no destination in mind. As you enter the traffic, since time is no problem—you don't need to rush anywhere—relax, slow down, and pay attention to all of the haste and craziness going on around you. You can observe it without being part of it. You are not battling to get ahead. If someone wants to break in front of you, slow down and let them. If someone is rude and aggressive, you don't care. Don't own their rudeness. Let it go. It is not part of your agenda. You are in the moment and focused on turning what would normally be "hassle time" into a real life version of ideal time—time where you take an activity that might be viewed as difficult or unpleasant (not unlike the challenges you will face visiting a friend with late stage Alzheimer's disease) and turn it around by going from a harried participant, caught up in the frenzy of the moment, into an observer, listening, present, and not judging.

Many people "run" from ideal time in that they establish such narrow boundaries that few actual experiences in their day-to-day lives qualify as ideal. Living in the moment and accepting the beauty and joy of consciously accepting that moment bring a special kind of peacefulness to your life. From this perspective, there should be no urgency to rush through what you are experiencing NOW (in the current moment), on the way to another more meaningful moment, because in rushing you lose sight of the meaning of what you are experiencing. Instead you are encouraged to be fully present and awake in the NOW. In the examples with my students, ideal is tied to enjoyment or comfort or familiar behaviors or memories. Ideal is about controlling our experience in

time to make it pleasurable. Unfortunately, as the students discovered, most of our everyday experiences don't fit this simple paradigm. As a result, the moments associated with ideal time can be very brief. However, when we expand our boundaries for ideal time to go beyond pleasure and include most experiences in our day, we stretch the joy we find in moments into much longer moments simply with this change in perception. Such long moments are the heart of our experience in the world. And it will come as no surprise that they are crucial in dealing with Alzheimer's disease.

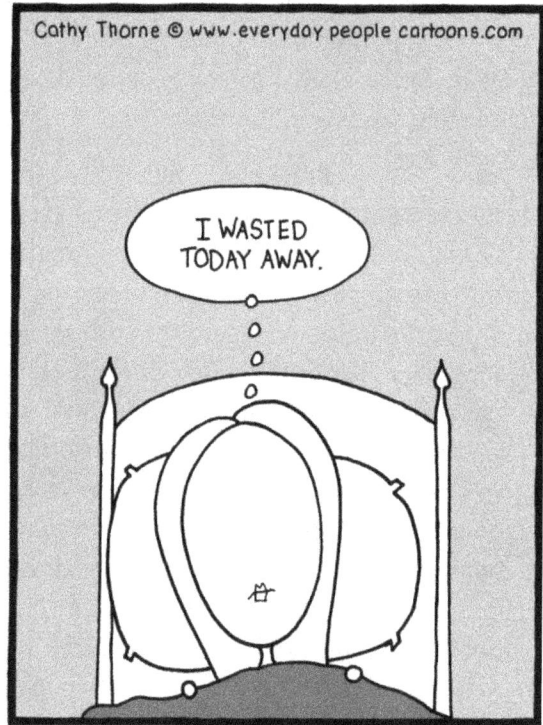

Cathy Thorne © www.everyday people cartoons.com

I WASTED TODAY AWAY.

BUT TOMORROW I PLAN TO BE PERFECT.

Imagine the difference in time spent with your friend or family member with Alzheimer's in these two scenarios. In Scenario 1 you are uncomfortable because you are not quite sure how to communicate with your friend and deal with their growing lack of connection to the world you once shared. In this case you are looking forward to the time when the visit or interaction is completed and you can go home or return to watching TV or cooking or whatever tasks would be part of your normal agenda. The bottom line here is that, defined in this manner, there is no ideal time or long moments when you are with your friend. There are only passing moments on the way to more familiar "turf" in your everyday patterns of living. Now consider Scenario 2 where, understanding the meaning of ideal time, you accept fully the responsibility of being in the moment with your friend. Just as in the example with rush hour traffic, you are not concerned about where you will be in the next hour. Instead, you are fully committed to making this time during your visit ideal time by listening, not hurrying, and enjoying what unfolds with some detachment and possibly even some amusement in the same sense you might be entertained by any person, child or adult, dealing with a world that doesn't always work the way they expected. This is the key to adding precious long moments. Your attention is tuned to the NOW, not the past or the future. As you will see in chapter 7, this approach opens many doors to healthy, fulfilling, loving interactions and quietly relieves you of much stress and uncertainty. Of course you are uncertain. No big deal, when your mind is in the present.

In this book I will describe Alzheimer's and a process for communicating with your friend or loved one suffering from this disease. My analogies about dreaming or other planets will at times make the process sound benign, as if poking this person with a stick could suddenly make them return to this reality in the fullest sense, or, as if visiting another planet in your mind is analogous to daydreaming. Unfortunately, nothing could be further from the truth. Alzheimer's is a progressive, insidious, disabling disease that is frustrating and terrifying to experience as the patient and often difficult, aggravating, and heartbreaking for the caregiver. But, regardless of where you are in this process, at the beginning, middle, or ending stages, like the students described above, you as the caregiver have choices to make about time.

If a "good day" with your friend is one where they remember you or can temporarily share your current consensual reality (where you both remember and agree on how to interpret the events of the world so you share similar visions of this world), then you are headed down the same well-intentioned but foolish path as the students who defined ideal time as pleasure. Most of the moments that you share with your friend will not fit this ideal paradigm any more than the idea that work or housecleaning is always fun. However, if the notion of "ideal" comes from a place where you are listening to the world and accepting what is given to you in the moment, not attempting to force it in the directions that bring you comfort and pleasure, and not objectifying and judging your friend with Alzheimer's, then you have a good chance of expanding your loving connection and support by adding many new shared long moments. The greatest gift you can bring your friend is the long moments, listening, not judging, with you fully present and engaged in the process of making all of the time you are there as ideal as possible.

The reality is that you will not always be comfortable, you may feel more frustrated than loving, and the familiar behaviors and patterns that in the past have connected you with your friend will often not be relevant. This is a time of uncertainty where what to say and what to do will often not be obvious. Your friend is on a journey, one that at this time in our medical reality is not reversible. They cannot come to you. You must reach out to them with the greatest gift of all, your time and love, focused on the present and delivered as long moments.

Chapter 1: The Long Moment

Life is little more than a fleeting set of moments, dancing shadows on a wall that fade and disappear as a cloud crosses the sun or castles in the sand that transform and vanish with each new tide. All of the events of our lives, all of our play, our work, our achievements are ultimately rolled up into these moments: some painful, some filled with joy, some so poignant they stay with us forever, but most go unnoticed and unacknowledged in our daily routines. They are the quiet now that forms the background of human consciousness. We live life in these brief moments anchored by our work, our play, our friends and families, and most of all by the habits and conventions we have adopted as our agreements with the universe. It is these agreements that allow us to operate, with little conscious effort, on auto-pilot for most of the time.

What is perhaps most special about these moments and at the same time largely taken for granted is that they are shared. They can be shared directly as you enjoy dinner at a cafe in Paris, a sunset on the ocean, a football game on TV, or driving to work in rush hour on a Los Angeles freeway with your friend or spouse. They can also be shared indirectly as you thrill me with the tales of your adventures in Africa on the last safari, bore me with the details of your clients' problems from work, or warm my heart with a story that touches your own emotions and feelings and mine. Directly or indirectly we live in the same world and through a combination of agreements between us, our educational system, our media, and the social reinforcement we give each other for sharing, openness, communicating, and connecting, we tune our minds to the same wavelengths within this universe. You see "red," I see "red." You see love, hate, kindness, injustice: I will typically see the same.

> *Dad planned his life with the expectation that he might get Alzheimer's disease (as did his father). Fortunately this never happened. On the night that he died, I spent several hours talking with him as his blood pressure slowly dropped from low to very low to the point where he lost consciousness. Our last moments were filled with his concerns over leaving Mom, his readiness to pass, and many, many stories and memories of events we shared together as a family and as friends. In our time together, we had many long moments, but none more precious than those remembered and shared at the end.*

No, we don't always agree, but even when we disagree, we are always still in agreement about the underlying rules and boundaries that guide our perception of reality and that make politics or fine art or beauty or social behavior possible. Our agreements exist and take on meaning because these underlying agreements about social reality are in place. This is not always the case when you enter another culture and some of our shared conventions are no longer as important. In most modern cultures today, certainly Western cultures, the power of "me" or "I" dominates our thinking, whereas in many native cultures the "we" or "us" dimension is much stronger. My friend and business partner in Russia reminds me that there is justice as we think of it in the United States and then there is justice as he (and much of the rest of the world) knows it. If you are arrested in his country, you are by definition guilty, not innocent until proved guilty.

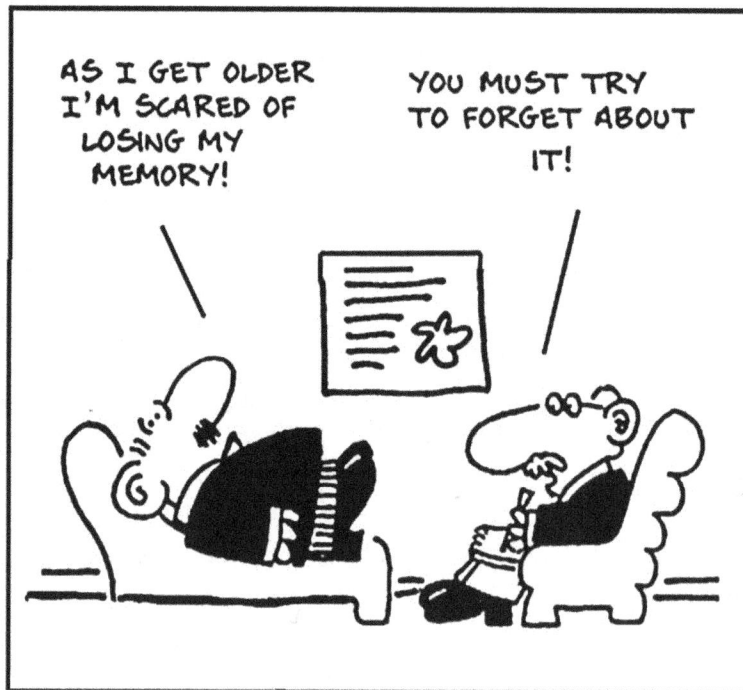

The agreements between us take place at several levels:

- **The verbal level (conscious)**: We understand and can communicate about many things in the world, the history, the cost, the size, the color, our likes and dislikes, and a thousand other factors. This level is largely about self-talk (what we say to ourselves) and our conversations with others.

- **The image level (conscious)**: Think of this as the right brain with its preference for images, holistic perceptions, and communication by pictures rather than words. Because words may speak much louder than images in our mind, the presence of right-brain consciousness may not be obvious to us.

- **The auditory level (conscious and unconscious)**: Sounds other than speech often represent images or holistic perceptions. Such sounds have a special meaning in the context of Alzheimer's disease. A favorite tune, for example, can be remembered even in the late stages and be a source of joy or, with the Alzheimer's Cards (discussed later), anchor a communication process.

- **The emotional/feeling level (conscious and unconscious)**: We understand and can share many emotions, love, anger, attraction, disappointment, and dozens more. They can be shared actively with words or gestures or more passively or be unconscious. The heart of the agreements at this level is our willingness to communicate and share feelings.

- **The physical or kinesthetic level (conscious and unconscious)**: This is the dimension of touch and special kinds of physical interactions that become part of our agreements, such as hugging, holding hands, kissing, and many other forms of affection. These agreements are especially important in dealing with Alzheimer's because many will be maintained as the disease progresses.

- **The background level (partially conscious)**: The majority of our agreements exist here and have become such a part of our habits and everyday perceptions that we normally don't need to think about them: colors, sounds, shapes, tastes, core sensations, much of nature, etc. My description of this level is oversimplified since many layers of consciousness that feed our agreements about reality lie beneath the surface of everyday reality. They are not unconscious, but like dreams or memories, they only emerge in our conscious mind when summoned.

- **The unconscious level (not conscious)**: Human consciousness exists on many planes simultaneously and just because our mind is not aware of something in the conscious realm does not mean we are not aware. It just means that we don't have conscious access to this memory most of the time. The unconscious is a vast domain that ranges from measureable acts of precognition (where a particular unconscious bias or predisposition can dramatically impact current perceptions) to elusive, mysterious dream states, meditative states, or biofeedback states that permit control over our autonomic systems through hypnosis or focused learning.

The core conflicts that feed the anxiety of an individual with Alzheimer's disease and family members or friends are often conflicts between conscious and unconscious perceptions of the world. On the caregiver side, for example, consciously you may feel a strong obligation to visit and support your spouse who has middle to late stage Alzheimer's and has entered a treatment facility that provides twenty-four-hour support. Unconsciously, you may still be upset because all of your life plans together and your personal plans are on indefinite hold as the disease progresses. On the patient's side, especially in the later stages of Alzheimer's disease, he or she may not consciously recognize the photo in front of them or the characters in the story you are telling, but the unconscious mind absolutely remembers these things, and the conflict produced, between what was remembered and what the person knows they should have remembered, is the origin of much frustration.

One important purpose of this book is, through stories and examples, to help you understand this conscious/unconscious conflict and find ways to bring the two minds together. Conscious/unconscious conflicts are very common in many life settings. As a sport psychologist, I would frequently see that consciously an athlete would be doing all they could to succeed, practicing, learning the sport, working hard, competing, while, at the same time, unconsciously, they were sabotaging the conscious goals with a lack of real interest or enthusiasm for the sport. This could show up as a fear of succeeding or with self-defeating statements such as "I really don't belong on this team." The parallel in health-related settings would be to consciously do healthy things to address a serious illness but unconsciously be producing the illness out of fear or a negative attitude about self ("I deserve to be sick").

At any stage in the Alzheimer's process, such conflicts can occur. The biggest clue is that when your conscious mind and unconscious mind are out of synch things don't feel right. When this happens, it is a warning signal that the two minds are not aligned and that it is worth pausing for a mo-

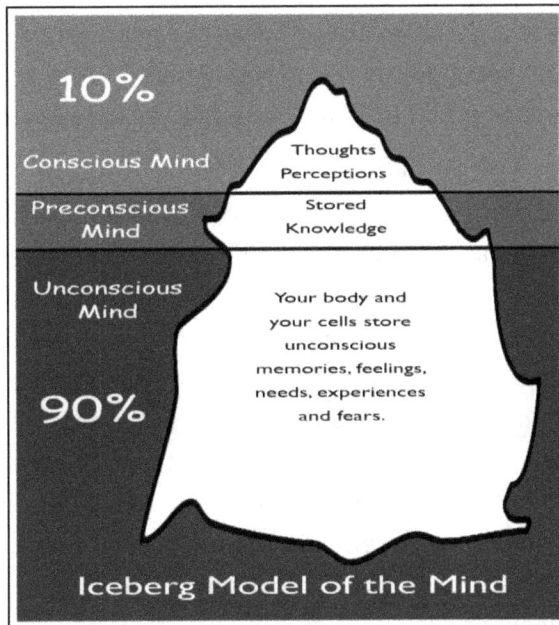

Iceberg Model of the Mind

ment to try and understand why. Usually it is the unconscious mind that "wins" these conflicts. You can continue to force yourself down the path that the conscious mind wants to pursue, but your unconscious will be relentless in producing symptoms that let you know the conflict exists and needs to be resolved, until you do reach resolution. Often these conflicts will be manifest as illness, exhaustion, general discomfort, or, in the case of an Alzheimer's patient, frustration and anger. If you are listening, a part of your mind will be screaming at you to wake up and pay attention.

Imagine the messages that are bouncing around in the mind of your friend or family member now as they begin a journey with Alzheimer's disease: confusion, fear, frustration, love, and an acceptance and understanding that they are traveling a one-way street with no exits and where, over time, the landmarks in this world they share with you will become progressively grayer, like walking into a fog that thickens with each step. Given the challenges along this path, where traditional forms of communication may be difficult, can you expect to find channels that will play the same message in both the conscious and unconscious theaters? As you read the chapters and stories that follow, look for the anchor agreements that are highlighted. Each of these agreements represents a communication channel, such as touch or memory of key life experiences or skills, which is almost always open as the disease progresses and which is likely to play the same tune both consciously and unconsciously. Think of a favorite song or melody from your past and your reactions as it is played. There is little doubt your cognitive, conscious reaction and the many possible unconscious reactions are in synchrony.

As your world and the world of your friend or partner begin to diverge, you will depend more and more on these alternate communication channels and less and less on the social agreements that dominate our everyday consciousness in Western society. I would love to be able to say that the new world that is emerging for your friend is a benign world that can comfortably replace the world they are leaving, the world they share with you. Unfortunately that is not the case, for entering this new world comes with the same anxieties you might feel entering the wilderness in a strange country where you do not understand the rules, what plants or animals are friend or foe, and what to expect in most communication, and, unfortunately living with Alzheimer's is about as benign as floating in a swimming pool filled with sharks. Even though, as you will see, your friend's world is still full of opportunities for love and laughter and richness from many long moments, given a choice, this is not a world they would ever enter voluntarily. That is the bad news. The good news is that this is life and like all dimensions of your life and your friend's life, it is filled with challenges, pain, and pleasure, and the glass is always half full just waiting for you to embrace that discovery with your friend in new ways.

It is true that at some point in the future your friend will be a stranger to you and you a stranger to them. In a half-empty worldview your relationship with them ends on a very sour note as this threshold is reached. This is not the choice you will make, correct? You will see the glass as half full and, as I describe in chapter 8, take the steps needed to meet this stranger, embrace their reality, and join them again as a friend.

If, in your own mind, as the person with Alzheimer's, you define a quality life as one where you continue to share the same reality that you always shared with friends, or, as the caregiver, you have a similar view, you

14

are bound to be disappointed. And once you start down this path and set up expectations in your mind with your self-talk, or conversations with yourself, it is difficult to stop. The message to hear now, in the beginning, is that the world has changed. You and your friend with Alzheimer's are less and less sharing the traditional world or reality that you are both used to, with its rich memory of shared experiences, its emphasis on evaluation and verbal behavior, and its continuity in time that allows you to connect today with yesterday and tomorrow in a meaningful sequence so that in any one moment your mind can be dealing with the present but feeding in data from your past and plans for the future, and more and more you are now sharing a world defined by the moments, in the present tense, when you are together.

At the beginning of the Alzheimer's process, with this mental shift in expectations, you have at least ten thousand long moments left to be with your friend. Yes, it is true that many of these moments will not be in your familiar, shared Earth-reality because that is a door that is closing quickly. But, that misses the point. If you care for your friend and your intention is add as much quality to the life of your friend as possible, you now have a path to follow to accomplish this. The idea is pretty simple. *You bring as much love and joy and quality to each of these ten thousand long moments as possible.* That is your focus, that is your goal, and that is the heart of the message I have to offer you in this book.

In chapters 6 and 7 we will see that in the middle and late stages of Alzheimer's disease the past and future largely disappear from the conscious mind. There is only NOW, in the moment. If in your visits with your friend you reach back into the past to try and rekindle memories and connections that are meaningful to you, the result will be to diminish the quality of this moment on this visit because your friend is living in the present and your testing of them will only lead to anxiety and frustration, not the gift you intended, I am sure. As you will see in chapter 4, it is often difficult to be clear and honest with yourself about the "why" of your visit. Is this visit really about you, not your friend with Alzheimer's disease? And if so, are you comforted when your friend remembers you and past experiences in their life with you? Or is this visit about them and your desire to bring comfort and love and meaning to as many long moments with them as possible? We will see!

As you sit and wait for the doctor and feel your partner's anxiety and your own, relax. You don't control or own the outcome. It is not your responsibility to fix things or make things right for your friend or loved one. You are surrounded by a universe filled with love, from God, from your friend, from the physicians and other treatment personnel, and from countless other sources that you cannot imagine. You are not responsible for the present circumstances. But you can choose to be a great friend or partner by accepting what is happening and deciding from this point on to share with them as many long moments as possible in whatever form they appear, in a familiar shared reality here on Earth or in parallel realities on different planets, it doesn't matter.

You would never criticize a friend for dreaming, as it is a state as natural as eating, talking, or playing. That is what is happening now. It matters little whether you are reading this at the beginning or middle or ending of the dream—your friend's dream is underway. I sincerely hope that the ideas and stories in this book help you become part of that dream, for as long as this is possible, and to preserve and enjoy many precious long moments of that dream together.

In many of the chapters that follow, I describe the experiences of the person with Alzheimer's with a *left-brain* perspective and also a *right-brain* perspective. Since these terms have so many meanings in the popular literature, it might be helpful to define them here. *Left brain* refers largely to the self-talk dimension of consciousness. Self-talk goes on constantly in our mind and is usually focused on the verbal, logical, linear (or step-by-step) aspects of reality. It is in this left-brain dimension where the first signs of Alzheimer's will appear as mistakes in memory or a breakdown in a common, everyday pattern that is tied to social interactions or everyday living (such as putting on pants before going outside or remembering why the frozen dinner is sitting on the kitchen counter). Along with the left brain comes what is perhaps the most emotionally discouraging aspect of Alzheimer's in the early stages and that is *evaluation*. The left brain is constantly measuring and "scoring" how well you are doing in the world, how people are reacting to you, or how competent you are in everyday tasks or your professional roles. As these processes experience some disruption in the early stages, it is difficult for friends and family not to evaluate and criticize or comment on problems the Alzheimer's patient is experiencing. It is also difficult for the patient not to be evaluating their own performance negatively, and the first place this will appear will be in the form of negative self-talk. ("What is wrong with me?" or "Why don't I remember his name?")

Right-brain consciousness is more tied to images or pictures and a holistic view of the world. It is always present in your mind, but it is often dominated by the noisy, talking left brain. It has been compared to the inside of a theater while the left brain is outside in the bright sunlight. When you enter the theater, you really cannot see very much because your eyes haven't adjusted to the reduced light. It often takes some practice with a discipline such as meditation to access this right-brain state of mind. To an Alzheimer's patient, the right-brain consciousness is extremely important because it is the gateway to many of the communication channels that remain open through the course of the disease, images of loved ones, patterns of daily routines, agreements and understandings about the world that can be shared. Your friend or family member may not know your name but they will recognize you. They may not remember the details of the cycling trip you took through Europe but they will remember the physical experience of cycling. Why is right-brain consciousness more robust here? Research suggests that images and holistic perceptions are less prone to disruption, at least in the early stages of Alzheimer's, because they represent patterns of neural activity that are less location-specific in the brain and can be accessed through multiple pathways, whereas a specific left-brain idea such as a name, place, or other specific detail tied to memory may no longer be accessible when a few key pathways are disrupted. The information is still present in the mind, just not available.

As the left brain begins to lose touch with the agreements that are part of your shared reality, look for opportunities to recover some of this communication ability through the right-brain channels of imagery, life experiences, skills, touch, and holistic memories. Each of these channels touches many dimensions of life, not just a few specific details such as a name or place. These other dimensions are elaborated on in several later chapters.

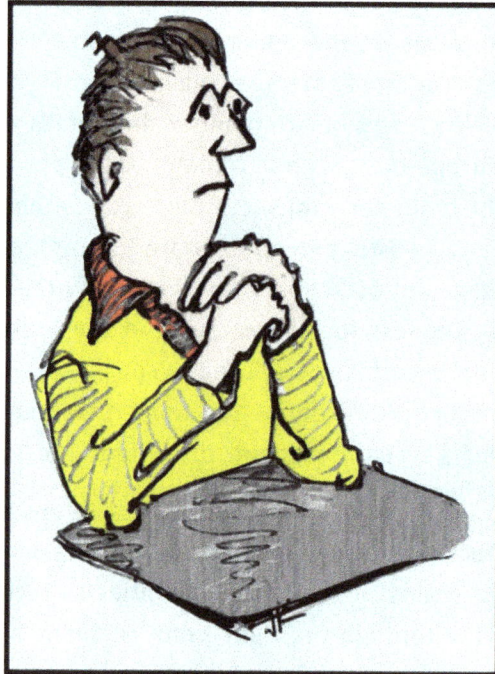

I have something to say!

Chapter 2: Hear My Voice

While on the surface this book is written for all of the parties involved with a person who has Alzheimer's disease, the family, the friends, the caregivers, the physicians and counselors, because this is the most likely audience, at its heart it is for and about that individual living with the disease. It is, in my limited way, an interpretation of their voice, of their frustration with our myopic view of their reality, of their needs, and of their desire to communicate, while we continue to fumble with a social reality that is no longer relevant to them. If you are "fortunate" to be in the early stages of Alzheimer's disease and reading this book and creating your Alzheimer's Cards in collaboration with your caregivers, my limitations will be even more obvious. I can no more be "in your world" than you can return to mine healthy and whole, but while we have time together, with your blessing and cooperation, perhaps we can lay the foundation for knowledge and tools to enhance your peace of mind and ability to communicate in the later stages.

I have briefly described the differences between left- and right-brain consciousness and how Alzheimer's patients gradually lose the ability to function well in a "left-brain" world that is dominated by linear, verbal, sequential thoughts and behaviors. This is a world that is validated every day through our agreements with each other about the meaning of things we collectively experience, going all the way from simple agreements about colors or shapes to more complex agreements about attitudes, behaviors, politics, and other social or ethical considerations.

While living in this shared reality, our ability to voice our intentions, our needs, our feelings, and most other personal requirements that give us a measure of control and competence on the planet Earth is strong. We can choose to have a loud voice or a quiet one, be passive or aggressive in meeting our needs, but, regardless, our ability to communicate clearly is always present. This voice speaks externally as we operate with proficiency in the world to control and manage parts of it as needed. It also drives us internally as our self-talk guides our every step and gives us a point of self-reference so that we can be simultaneously experiencing life *and* watching ourselves experiencing life at the same time. Can you remember talking with a potential romantic partner and at the same time you are talking be wondering how they are perceiving you? That type of self-referral process goes on continuously in our minds.

Alzheimer's disease changes the rules here dramatically and very quickly. When short-term memory and the logical/linear functioning of the brain suffers interference, normal behaviors taken for granted and guided by self-referral such as dressing or dining become problematic. Even worse, the communication of basic needs and thoughts becomes a process blurred by the impact that Alzheimer's has on typical speech and thought patterns, also dependent on self-referral. As the patient it is not so much that I cannot still communicate as the fact that once the familiar, left-brain, verbal/logical channels are compromised, the world on the receiving end of my communication is not prepared to listen through any other channel.

My Aunt Betty, mother's younger sister, was retarded and lived with my grandparents in Bolivar, Tennessee. When I was six, I shocked Mom one morning by asking what would happen to Betty when her parents died. Even as a child, I had noticed that her ability to function was challenged in some special ways. By the time I was a teenager, Betty was institutionalized and her weak voice already lost in the medicinal approaches to mental care common at the time. Mom complained after each visit that she seemed drugged and unresponsive and the combination of retardation and dementia rendered her helpless to the institution's protocol. I wondered what it would be like to be in Betty's situation, alive but helpless with no voice, lost in the bureaucracy of a "mental ward" in a state hospital.

This is one of the great frustrations of every individual who experiences the mental deterioration that is part of the Alzheimer's disease process. As the patient, you have a lot more say than your family, your friends, or your caregivers are prepared to receive. Prior to Alzheimer's, your internal voice is clear: "Hi, my name is Rich and I am trying to take a nap. All that noise you are making is disturbing me!" Now try that same statement when the internal voice can no longer be separated into a part that is talking and another part that is listening (self-referral). "I am upset" is one possible outcome. I have lost the ability to take an experience (the noise) and convert it into an abstract version of the experience (I say to myself that it is very noisy) and then connect that to an emotion (I am upset). This process no longer works. In the simplest terms, you have "lost your voice."

Imagine with me for a moment how you will change as the disease progresses. In the early stages, the communication process is largely normal as

20

you are forgetting things, but logical, linear thinking guided by self-talk still dominates your consciousness. This communication process is likely to be confounded with the presence of the diagnosis of Alzheimer's in your life and the ripple that causes with family, friends, and future plans. Nevertheless, when you need to communicate and plan, you are able to be clear about your needs, to yourself and others. At some point in the future, however, you will begin to have difficulty with behaviors that define the basic patterns of everyday life, such as dressing, preparing meals, going to the store, taking a walk outside, and so forth. Even at this stage, however, you are likely to both understand the problems you are having and have a voice in working out the best solution. Now jump to the stages where very little of your time is spent in our shared Earth-reality and the people in your life who represent your significant others have become strangers. What is your voice like now? In our left-brain, verbal world, it's a weak voice. While you can still recognize words and sentences and understand them, they have little connection with you because your self-talk no longer references the abstract "you" that is the subject of the talk. It is a giant leap to go from reading the words "I am hungry" to the self-referencing required to connect these words to a need state in your body. Others are making all of the decisions for you. Other than expressing yourself emotionally or physically, it is difficult to communicate. And in the later stages of Alzheimer's disease that will follow the voice will diminish even further.

By this time the world is not expecting very much from you. You are present physically, but for all practical purposes, you are no longer sharing the same reality, correct? After all, what could you say about anything in your life that would be accepted as a comment from the real you versus a comment distorted by the you with an Alzheimer's mind? Not much. Part of the problem here is our limited understanding of the nature of human consciousness. We experience the world largely through the filter of the verbal/logical left brain and the constant conversations in our head as we "talk to ourselves." When this logical, talking world is shut down, our consciousness and shared perceptions of the world to a large degree also shut down.

But not completely. Certainly when the part of our mind that controls the centers for speech and logical thinking is damaged, these functions are damaged, but human consciousness is much more complex and multidimensional than we would expect based on our day-to-day experience. It actually operates on many layers simultaneously, but these layers are not part of our awareness because left-brain, talking, controlling consciousness is so dominant. Our experience of life, our memories, feelings, and perceptions, are all represented in this set of other dimensions of consciousness, and are all opportunities for communication.

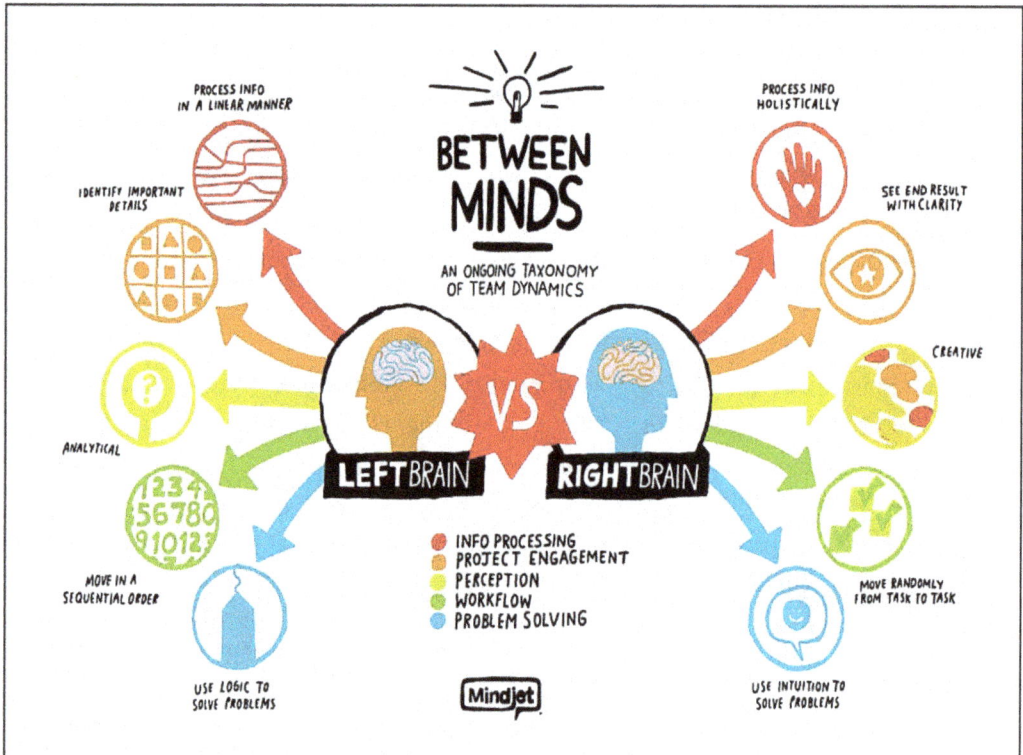

Right-brain functions are less impacted by Alzheimer's.

The key point here is that most of these dimensions will continue to be channels for communication and reasoning long after our shared left-brain consciousness has been compromised. In other words, not only is there a place to look to find your voice but we can also expect that voice to connect to many parts of your consciousness that are relatively intact.

Now when we ask the question, do you have anything to say about your choices in the mid and late stages of Alzheimer's disease, when our shared realities no longer intersect, the answer is, of course, yes. But, in the same way that hearing-impaired individuals need a hearing aid to amplify sounds or most of us need glasses or contacts as adults, cognitively impaired individuals with

Alzheimer's need their own kinds of aids to help filter their true "voice" from the noise and confusion generated by the brain. The Alzheimer's Cards described in Appendix A are one such tool.

Look at the image in the illustration on page 24. If you move your eyes close to the full-size image, the face disappears, leaving only the lines. When you back up and view the image from a distance, the face appears! Imagine for a moment that the close view here is similar to having a typical, left-brain conversation with an Alzheimer's patient. While the speaker operates at a normal social level filling the conversation with details, about memories, today's experiences, the people who are present, the environment, the food, and so forth, the listener is operating at a more holistic level and only in the present tense. The result is that the voice of the speaker will miss its intended target; hence, the attempted conversation is likely to be stressful and not especially meaningful to both caregiver and patient.

When you view the image from a distance, immediately you have a different perspective. Because the details are no longer dominating your vision, you can clearly see the overall pattern, the face. Many kinds of memories are stored in this manner, not as specific details but as patterns or holistic concepts. Much research and practical experience from those living and working with Alzheimer's patients supports this basic idea: Information that is distributed holistically across the brain (think of a pattern or concepts rather than details) is less impacted by Alzheimer's disease. Experiential memory of major life events or specific kinesthetic behaviors, such as riding a bike, have this property in many cases.

Why are these kinds of memories less impacted by Alzheimer's than memory of a specific short-term event, such as what you had for breakfast? Short-term memories tend to reside in one or two areas of the brain, the visual cortex and the speech centers located in the left hemisphere. To become long-term memories, even a memorable event such as a surprise birthday party with dancing bears, takes time and repetition to consolidate, encode, and store so that it can be recalled at a later time. This is not going to happen to individuals with Alzheimer's disease. Instead the memory is being distorted by the disease even as it is temporarily stored in a temporary location in the mind. When the question "What did you have for breakfast?" is asked an hour (or even a few minutes) later, the memory (a) may no longer exist in the mind, (b) may no longer be recognizable, or (c) may not be accessible because the neural connections between the "question" and the "information about breakfast" no longer exist. And, by the way, who was this abstract person that had breakfast!

At the same time the conscious mind is struggling with the question about breakfast and how to access this memory that quite possibly no longer exists in a recognizable form, much of the rest of your consciousness is not struggling, but, alas, these other layers are, for the most part, not accessible. Your body knows that it had breakfast. The visual and kinesthetic experience of having breakfast is likely to be stored not as a unique experience but part of a

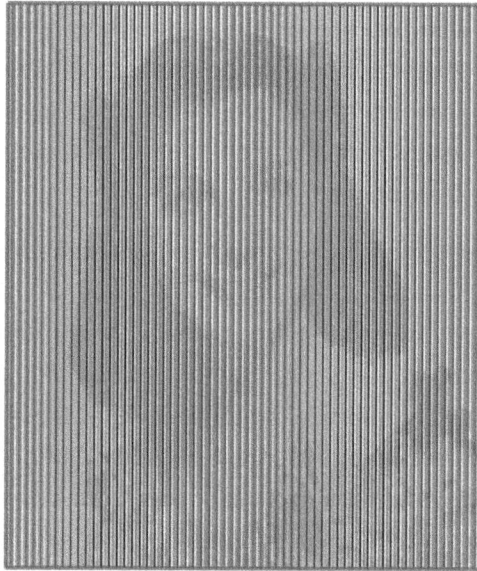

Think big picture. It is not about the details!

familiar pattern of experiences, like riding a bike, that are associated with waking up and beginning the day. At a deeper level, you are processing not just "having breakfast" but having breakfast in the context of how you feel physically and mentally, your level of confusion or clarity in the moment, who was in the room with you, and whether the experience conformed to a normal pattern or one that differed in a good or bad manner.

For example, what would happen if I showed a photograph of your plate at breakfast? Or, what if I place a set of cards on the table with images of eggs, coffee, cereal, orange juice, pancakes, etc. and asked you to connect them with the word "BREAKFAST." What we would learn is that our friend with Alzheimer's has a great deal more information stored than our original conversation would suggest—information about everything, breakfast, the past day,

24

their life with you, their care at home or in the treatment facility. The problem is that they cannot share it with you using conventional, conversational means.

Then, of course, there is the complexity added by a corrupted internal clock. Middle and late stage Alzheimer's patients live in the present, period. There is no past, no future, only the present tense is available. Ironically, patients in these stages have reached a true Zen-like state where they live consciously only "in the moment." In our conversational, left-brain Earth-reality, however, we juggle the present, past, and future simultaneously in our minds and, of course, expect others to understand us as we jump from the present tense to the future subjunctive to the hypothetical past! And, unfortunately, because Alzheimer's patients are not anchored to the continuum of time, left alone without our intervention, their moments in the present can repeat, over and over.

Now you can see the heart of the matter. Not only "am I still here" but my voice that can connect with you and through this connection share with you some of my needs and intentions "is still here." The catch is, as the patient, you have to come to me, in the moment in the present tense. I cannot come to you. There will be hundreds of opportunities for you to add quality to my life by making the moments we spend interacting meaningful, grounded in my present reality, and guided by the tools and techniques that work for my Alzheimer's consciousness.

In chapter 4, I will describe an important set of communication tools that take advantage of the power of these holistic, nonverbal layers of consciousness to help keep the voice in the Alzheimer's patient's mind open and communicating. In most of the chapters that follow, there will be a section called "Hear My Voice" in an attempt to speak to and for the individual suffering from Alzheimer's disease.

HEAR MY VOICE
The Alzheimer's Cards

My Dear Friend or Loved One,

As my Alzheimer's disease progresses, as you know, normal conversations will become more and more difficult because the speech centers in my brain and other functions that tie to short-term memory and linear, logical thinking will be impacted. Much of my mind and my experience (conscious and unconscious) will be impacted much more slowly by the disease. However, the problem will be that there are no communication channels for me to reach out to you with my awareness and intentions. I will still want to make some choices in my life and be capable of doing so but not able to communicate my needs!

To help me communicate, I need a language that works across many layers of consciousness, in the moment, and also has meaning for both of us. The language we create will need to be very direct and clear. It can also use images and be symbolic in ways that connect to details in my life that will always have meaning. Think of learning to ride a bike or music that I love or when I was married. These experiences will still be present in my mind long after normal speech and my memory of you as my spouse or friend have gone.

What I need for you to do is to help me find or create a personal set of Alzheimer's Cards that is appropriate for my current stage. In the early/middle stages the cards may connect to the important events and people in my life and have complex images or words associated with them. In the later stages I may need very simple cards with few words and limited (or no) images to represent each crucial area for communication. Appendix A gives additional information on the cards. Instructions on how to create and use the deck are included in the companion book, *The Alzheimer's Cards: Hear My Voice.* In chapter 7 are some examples of how the deck can be used to communicate with you when my everyday voice in Earth-reality is gone.

As you will see, the cards are one of the last bridges I will have between my shared world with you on Earth and the new planet, Altzair, where as a person with Alzheimer's, I reside.

Thank you for your love and support!

Chapter 3: The Diagnosis

It has been a very long morning. Mom and I spent most of it sitting in the waiting room of the Jefferson Clinic as Dad has gone back and forth for a variety of physical and mental tests. Finally we are all together in Dr. Blackstone's office waiting for his evaluation.

Dr. Blackstone: "I know this is not the news you wanted but after looking at the test results it is fairly certain that Frank is showing the symptoms of early stage Alzheimer's. Physically he is very healthy and at sixty-two I think we can rule out most other forms of dementia due to aging, plus the tests and his behavior the last few months are more indicative of Alzheimer's disease."

Even though this was expected, we collectively sigh with disappointment and Mom leans across to Dad and hugs him for a few seconds. Dad's face is drained of color and I can hear his breathing quicken as each inhalation becomes a gulp.

"There are a number of things we can do to slow the onset of the disease. There are some promising new medicines and the latest research has suggested some mental exercises that can help delay the onset of some symptoms, but, at the moment, as you know, there is no available treatment that can stop or reverse the progression of the disease and over time you can expect the symptoms to increase. Modern medicine has advanced in so many areas but Alzheimer's is still largely a mystery. We cannot offer a cure or even predict how quickly the disease will develop. It is a day-by-day process."

Frank: "So I will just get worse and worse, right?"

"Yes and no. Physically you are likely to continue with a normal, slow aging process for many years. Mentally, the symptoms you are experiencing now, the gaps in time during the day, not remembering friends, places, or why you are doing a specific task, and your frustration, all of these will worsen over time. How rapidly, we cannot say for sure. As the disease advances, you can expect symptoms that will include confusion, irritability, and aggression, some of which you are already experiencing. Also it is not uncommon for sufferers to withdraw from family and friends in general at some point."

"Not fun. How long do I have?"

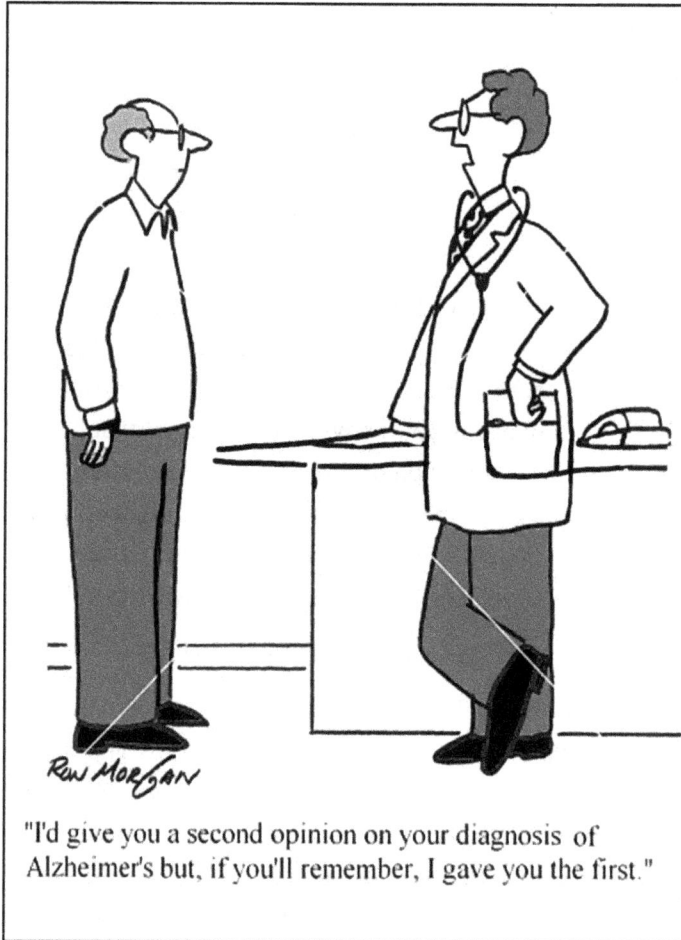

"I'd give you a second opinion on your diagnosis of Alzheimer's but, if you'll remember, I gave you the first."

"That is hard to say. Since the disease is different for each individual, predicting how it will affect you as a person is difficult. Life expectancy following diagnosis is typically six to eight years but a very small percentage of people will live ten to twelve years."

"Will Dad need to be hospitalized?"

"Perhaps, this is an option to consider at some point. For many families this is just not practical. However, now, in this early stage, it is likely that Frank can live several years with you at home if your lifestyle allows you or other family members to be home with him, when needed, as caregivers. With the exception of some of the memory and behavior problems that Frank is currently experiencing, he will feel and think and act normally. In the later stages, Alzheimer's is known for placing a huge burden on caregivers and, at some point, he will begin to need full-time care in order to function safely since many of the things we take for granted today—meals, cleaning, walking outside, interacting with friends—will be challenging for your dad. For his safety and comfort, you will want some help here and our experience suggests that being with him every day may be more stressful than helpful."

I remember when Aunt Emilou was first diagnosed with Alzheimer's disease. She had been having trouble for several months, living alone in her apartment. Her daughter Katherine found her outside on the porch one day, in her nightgown, confused about why she was there. Several times, in the kitchen, she watched as Emilou would start to make a sandwich or coffee and end up halfway through the process not sure what to do next. She was losing weight, not bathing properly, not fixing her hair, and the apartment was a mess. That's when Katherine made the appointment to visit the clinic. We were thinking dementia but were not surprised to hear the doctor say it was definitely Alzheimer's disease.

I thought of Dad at the time and the irony of the fact that he worried constantly about Alzheimer's and had no problem while Emilou, with her busy, giving life never gave it a thought!

"Stressful ... for us? I guess we can expect that."

"Yes, it is very hard for a spouse or a child not to remember the way things were before Alzheimer's and to look for these things in visits and interactions. When something that was shared previously can no longer be shared, it can be quite frustrating both for you and for your dad. Remember that normally, as we live every day, we are constantly evaluating things. How does this taste? How good is this meal or book or TV show? Does that comment from a friend make sense?"

"Of course. We do constantly think about things and how we feel about them."

"Already, as you have described, that process can be the source of some frustration. On the one hand, you are hoping that today will be a day when everything is 'normal' and Frank is behaving like the person you have known for many years. Said another way, you are looking for these typical, familiar behaviors and *evaluating* whether or not they occur. This is not meant to be a negative act. We evaluate the world constantly. In fact, it is normal for visitors to say that a family member with Alzheimer's is 'having a good day' when they can share memories with you and act similar to what was experienced in the past. But, can you see how unfair that is?"

"Unfair, what do you mean?"

"Let me give you an example. If you sat down next to a close friend or family member and starting talking about your childhood or parents or other events in your life, you would expect them to remember and understand most of what your were saying. Correct?"

"Yes."

"But what about a stranger? Would you expect the stranger to remember these events and to share your experiences?"

"Of course not. But Dad is not a stranger. He may have Alzheimer's but he still remembers many of these experiences."

"But he doesn't remember all of them, even now in the early stages. In addition, these long-term memories are being compromised by the disruption in Frank's short-term memory where Alzheimer's is having the strongest impact. Over time he will lose the ability to connect with more and more of these memories. When you are with him, you remember another person, a person whose mind is clear and not impaired. You both will, for the rest of your lives, want to remember this person, the one who is your dad and your partner, not the one who is becoming a stranger. But you cannot stop the process that has started. Even at this moment, Frank is, in part, sitting in this room with us, listening and knowing that he is grateful to be here in the same world as the two of you and knowing that you love him, and in part he is already experiencing

30

the disconnect that comes from being in another world. As the disease progresses, he will, not by his own choosing, become more and more a part of this other world. In the clinic we call this other world the planet 'Altzair' to remind us that our patients really are experiencing a reality that is different that we cannot see or understand.

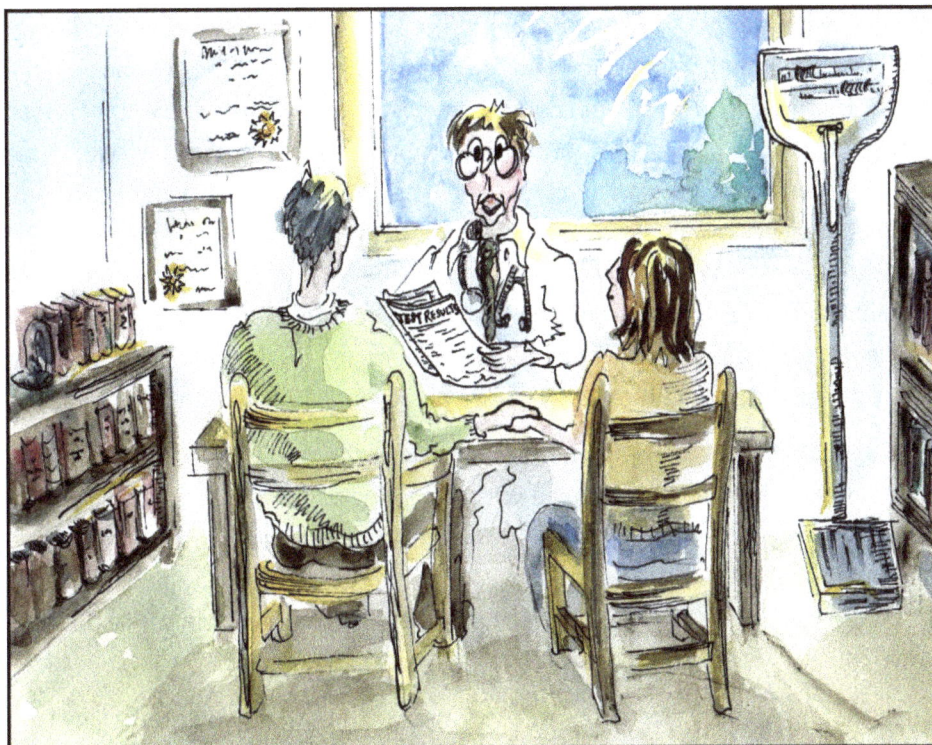

It is important to listen and not evaluate. That's how you can help to turn frustration into precious long moments.

Frank has been listening but shifting restlessly as Dr. Blackstone was speaking. Finally, he interrupts.

"You are right. It feels like another planet. One moment I am OK and the next my mind has zoned-out and is no longer connected with this world. It is very frustrating because I don't know when it will happen next or what to do when it does happen."

"If there were a simple bridge between Altzair and Earth that you could cross, you would do this in a minute, but generally you won't have this opportunity. You cannot take this step."

Dr. Blackstone turns to face me.

"So, despite your wishes and his, eventually he will be a stranger. His intentions and needs and your intentions and needs won't be aligned any more than you and a true stranger that you meet on the street are aligned. Now do you see my point? It's not fair for you to pressure him to cross that bridge back to your world and your memories when he cannot. It is also not fair for you to judge him by whether or not he can make that journey; he doesn't control this decision. If you want to define a 'good day' as one when he is able to connect with you, that is fine and is your choice. But for him a 'good day' won't be about this world or crossing a bridge to it to be with you. It is much more about living as peacefully as possible and enjoying his moments in life in an environment that is already very stressful and confusing. Please realize that the worst possible stress can come from you, someone he knows he has an emotional connection with, which he feels, but then does not understand why you are angry or frustrated with him."

Frank: "I know what you mean, Dr. Blackstone. It is difficult for me now, Julie, when you are upset with me in the morning as I try to get up, dress, and come to breakfast—and instead wander into the study and sit in front of the computer or wander outside. You don't mean to be annoyed, I know, but your frustration with me is pretty obvious and it makes me feel helpless and angry with myself."

"I'm so sorry. I don't mean for my frustration to show but I am frustrated. I love our life together and I don't want it to change."

"I know. Me either."

Dr. Blackstone: "There is still lots of living for the two of you and still many long moments together as well as apart. My advice to all of you is, 'don't waste them.' They are precious regardless of the form they take as shared moments in a world you all remember or as moments in separate worlds. As the Alzheimer's progresses, because we know so little about how to delay or stop that progression, more and more of Frank's experiences will be in his world, not one you can share with him. Research suggests that often he will be dreaming of your world and remembering things in this world that go all the way back to his childhood, but, like most dreams, while clear for a moment in his mind, they may not be real in any sense that could be communicated or shared with you.

He will be living on his own planet, Altzair, where the rules are different from those in Earth-reality.

"Frank is living in a kind of prison, one created completely by his mind, but a prison nevertheless, from which he cannot escape. It's a prison that will shut out his connections to the past and the future but leave him many long moments in the present. He needs your help to make his stay there as peaceful and loving and as connected to those who care for him as possible. That's your job. Today is the first day on that job. Eventually the Frank you know now will be a stranger to you and you will need to meet, accept, and embrace that stranger, but that is several years away. Finally, I know you will need some help not just from me but from many other health care professionals as well as your family and friends. We cannot reverse the path Frank is on, but seeing it many times, we have much to offer to support you, the caregivers, and to keep you healthy.

"Just three gentle reminders before you leave today. First, Alzheimer's is much like life because it will be with Frank until he dies, so enjoy every moment with him. Second, no matter how much frustration or anxiety you feel, for many years Frank will be feeling more. He is the one on the journey to an unknown place, and because it is his mind, he is there twenty-four/seven. Finally, we are so used to judging things in our lives that we take it for granted. Frank needs your love and unconditional acceptance, not your judgment. The game he is playing now is really about his comfort and his peace of mind. Both will become more and more precious. To help him the most, you will have to play by his rules, respecting his reality because he can never return to yours.

Grieving, Hospice, and Alzheimer's

In a healthy environment, a diagnosis of Alzheimer's disease is, in many respects, the beginning of the hospice process for both the caregiver and the patient. Yes, of course, the term *hospice* refers to a focus on "keeping the individual comfortable until death" rather than focusing on "keeping the individual alive as long as possible using medical interventions." So acknowledgment of death is part of your life's process as well. As a culture we tend to be squeamish about death and regard it as tragic only when it is unexpected or when it shortens an anticipated lifespan. Depending on the age of the person diagnosed with Alzheimer's that may or may not be the case.

The beauty of hospice is that it represents a formal acknowledgment that death at some point is inevitable and that what is important now is living comfortably not prolonging life in pain. What better way is there to describe the Alzheimer's process? In the late stages as both physical and mental functioning is seriously impacted, a traditional hospice process is often the best option for both patient and caregiver. In the early and intermediate stages, hospice has a different meaning. It does, of course, communicate that death is coming—no surprise here—but, more importantly, it speaks to how you, the caregiver, behave now. Your role is to bring comfort and peace. There is no medical intervention that can currently help, except in a temporary way. Bring peace and comfort. Listen, support, avoid judgment, trust in spirit, be fully present, and most of all, offer the gift of many long moments. That is the essence of hospice as it applies to Alzheimer's disease.

Grieving is a process that we often associate with hospice and death. But, of course, it is also very much a part of current life events. We can grieve for the loss of a job, a relationship, a home, a skill, our personal security, or many other aspects of our present existence in Earth-reality. In the case of Alzheimer's disease, it is natural to begin grieving over the loss of the expected normal life and aging process with a friend, spouse, or family member long before death occurs.

Just learning of the diagnosis of Alzheimer's disease can initiate many emotions: sadness, disappointment, fear, concern, longing, love, and a sense of helplessness as you face the inevitability of a proscribed future. It is natural and not unhealthy to shift mentally from anxiety about a possible diagnosis to grief about the consequences of the reality of that diagnosis. Learning of the diagnosis you may already begin to grieve the loss of your friend. It comes as a shock to our systems. It brings to mind our own vulnerability to disease and the prospect of our death. It can be emotionally devastating. How can you cope *and* be the strong, balanced, loving ally your companion needs as they too struggle with the implications of the diagnosis?

You will learn just as hospice caregivers learn, over and over, that true greatness is accessible to us all through our service to others. You will learn that patience, listening, quiet love, and sharing trump all active interventions that over the long run are doomed to failure. You will learn that the sense of grief you feel is not going to go away; it is part of the process of living with someone who has Alzheimer's disease. But this is OK. It is part of your process of living now. At times you may feel overwhelmed because once the grieving process begins, it is with you twenty-four/seven until at long last you are able to integrate the grief into your heart and let it become a part of you. Concentrate on the moments because that is where your friend is living. Make them long moments that comfort, stimulate, entertain, hear, and love your friend. That is your role. This is your mission as a caregiver and partner.

Remember that in offering kindness and love to your friend, you are really offering yourself the olive branch of peace. You are releasing the "what-ifs" of plans made in a life together and the anger you feel because this diagnosis will change your life in many ways that are not pleasant and not of your own choosing. Know that whatever happens you will find contentment for yourself through your acceptance of this diagnosis and your commitment of service to your companion.

Into the Gates of Hell

Imagine, for a moment, the experience of an Alzheimer's diagnosis in comparison to another, more familiar context, that of incurable cancer. Let's examine two different but similar situations.

Case 1: Your best friend has been diagnosed with incurable lung cancer. Those years of being a smoker have finally caught up with him. Your physician explains that with treatment and medication he will live for several more years but that death due to the cancer or its complications is inevitable.

Case 2: Your eight-year-old has been diagnosed with Alexander's disease, an incurable disease of the central nervous system. With treatment, he will live another two to three years with the symptoms and complications becoming worse over time.

My question for you to consider is, "How do you handle these two situations?" Obviously this is not good news. Obviously (assuming the physicians are correct) there is no hope for a cure and the impact of the disease on their lives will only worsen over time. Obviously, the specter of death and our personal and cultural issues with its significance looms over both situations. Obviously, there is a huge impact on finances, family, caregivers, life plans—all of the things we see with Alzheimer's disease.

But, as you consider these two sad but not uncommon scenarios and then think about our reaction to a diagnosis of Alzheimer's disease, there is a difference, isn't there? What is it? Alzheimer's has a mystique that is special and unique in an unfortunate way that makes it unlike any other disorder. It is this mystique that adds a special hopeless quality to the diagnosis. It also supports and maintains the cultural perception that the disease process is truly a "decent into hell." Let's see if we can understand the differences between the two cancer scenarios and the Alzheimer's scenario to get to the heart of the matter here.

Consider Case 1 where your friend has lung cancer. What do you do, beyond the normal reactions of grieving and preparing for their eventual death? Do you give up hope? Do you greet them with down-turned eyes and despair in your heart? Do you trivialize their approaching death by denying it? Do you treat them as less of a whole person because their life-clock has suddenly speeded up and their time on Earth, in this existence, has been shortened?

Of course not. Once you work through whatever grieving and denial is required after the diagnosis, you accept the reality of the present situation and deal with it. You make plans based on their eventual death. You concentrate on bringing joy and meaning to their life in the present even as you struggle with the concept of their eminent death. You bring care and comfort to them. Long moments with them take on a new meaning. You listen to their needs and struggles and fears and join them, if possible, in a real place where you are no longer advising or proscribing but just listening. In summary, you join the flow of the natural process that will lead inevitably from life today, before the diagnosis, through a series of transitions, to death.

But, you never, never, never give up hope. Hope is not about a miracle cure leading to recovery (unless you choose to be in denial). Instead, hope is about living a full life in a compressed time frame, joyfully, realistically, and without fear. This is the gift you bring with each visit, each plan, each action you take as a friend or loving partner.

Now consider Case 2 when the diagnosis is for a child. Much of the process is similar to Case 1 where grief and practical concerns and the concept of death are part of what is on your mind. But here there is also an important difference. Your friend with lung cancer most likely lived a "full life" or at least lived long enough so that the concept of death at the end of life is a natural and not unfamiliar consequence. This is not the same for a young child where death is much more of an abstraction. At age seven or eight, you are not concerned about living another eighty years, you are concerned about living now.

A child's perception of themselves with incurable cancer is simply that they are themselves and the cancer is an attribute, like braces, that causes some inconvenience but has little to do with who they are as a person. They are the same person. I don't mean to minimize the pain and discomfort that is part of the "inconvenience," but unless we tell them otherwise, they are alive, in the moment, waiting for us to guide them, love them, and support them. Having cancer may interfere with making the next Little League baseball practice but does not detract from that child's essence unless we, as adults, confound the two and overwhelm them with our sense of time and the tragedy about their short life. Why would we want to do that? Our intention for the child and for our loved one with Alzheimer's disease is for them to still experience hope, joy, and the fullness of life.

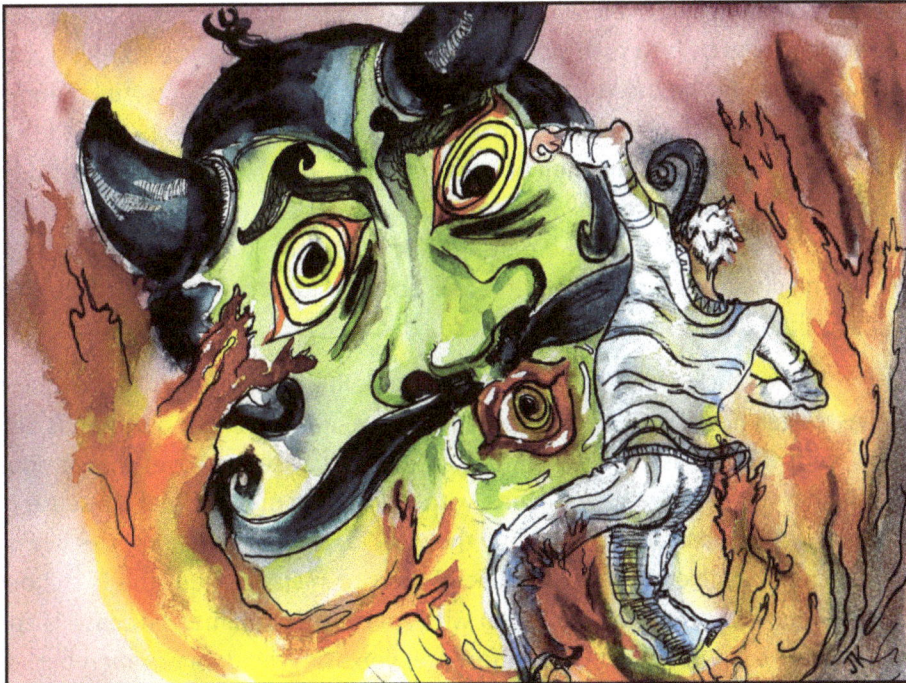

Battling the Alzheimer's Devil

Does it not surprise you that we would deny Frank the same grace that we routinely give others with terminal diseases even when many of these disorders lead to outcomes that are similar to Alzheimer's? Our perception of Frank is not that he is living his life fully and richly until the end, as in Case 1 above, or that he is the same person, just with Alzheimer's disease. Instead he is Frank with Alzheimer's disease lost in a hopeless and worsening cycle of mental and physical deterioration. With the diagnosis, he is literally standing at the gates of hell.

What is wrong with this picture? The answer is not that Alzheimer's disease is so insidious in its own special way that it is not comparable to other terminal diseases, even though it is obviously unique and does create its own special circumstances. The answer is that "we" are in the wrong here (or not in the light). Our culture and our medical establishment have taken the wrong approach in dealing with Alzheimer's disease. Inadvertently we dehumanize the symptoms of the disease, and out of fear of the unknown and unimaginable, the rules underlying our perception of reality are corrupted. We deny the Alzheimer's patient hope because we believe there is no hope. It is our fear and our uncertainty that block the offer of grace.

Imagine telling the child in Case 2 that he has no hope, that the cancer has changed who he is to such a degree that all he has to look forward to is a continuous decline in the quality of life with increasing pain, fear, and frustration—and by the way, in the later stages, communication will be so compromised that his family will not understand him or even recognize who he is. Sounds ridiculous, doesn't it? But this is essentially what we do with a diagnosis of Alzheimer's disease. Yes, there will be long moments and the descent will be gradual, but, of course, the disease is terminal and there is no hope for a cure. No, it is true that you have little to look forward to in life. Too bad.

While much of this last statement is certainly true, much of it is not, and the lies we tell here are lies of convenience for us, not to benefit our friends and family with the disease. Remembering Case 1 and Case 2 above, the obvious truth is that we want Frank or anyone with a diagnosis of Alzheimer's disease to live, fully, happily, and completely until they die. In all three situations, this will be difficult or impossible at times, because of the circumstances, but this is still our hope. In all three cases, the individual with cancer or Alzheimer's disease is still the same person with one crucial difference, you, the friend, family member, or caregiver. With cancer you can relate to the mind of the person with the disease and encourage them to share with you their condition, their feelings, and their needs. You can offer words of encouragement and hope and be there for them. You can support and be part of a "life lived fully" right until the end.

With Alzheimer's disease, there is a world of difference. Even in the early stages, the common ground of a shared reality and shared memories begins to suffer from gaps in communication. How can you live a full life when you can no longer communicate in the same language that is tied to your shared memories and experiences? How can life be full when a simple sequence of actions such as getting dressed or making a sandwich no longer is possible? In our culture today we don't have models or a language to describe this kind of disability. We are prepared to help you if you are "handicapped" in some of the proscribed, traditional ways, but not at all prepared when left-brain functions such as speech, logical sequences of behaviors, and a common understanding of the world around us are diminished.

Now you understand the problem and at least part of the solution. It is our job as friends, caregivers, health professionals, and society to accept the person diagnosed with Alzheimer's as the same person prior to the diagnosis. Just as a wheelchair changes our relationship with a family member in certain ways, Alzheimer's disease changes our relationship on different dimensions, but does not change the individual. Despite all the confusion and loss on so many levels, the essential nature of your friend or loved one with Alzheimer's remains. Living life fully has a different meaning for each individual in each situation. It is how we embrace handicaps brought on by disease, accidents, aging, or any of life's circumstances that counts. Alzheimer's disease is just another circumstance where we have to learn to accept, adapt, and join the flow. It is not a death sentence or a sentence to hell, although at times it may seem so.

It is our own fear and confusion tied to our dependency on the logical self-talk that runs through our mind from morning until night that limits the possibilities for the Alzheimer's patient. We are afraid because we control our world through this logical self-talk that guides our every behavior. When this self-talk and the associated memories are distorted, it in turn distorts our communication with others, which means, quite simply, that we are no longer sharing the same world. This loss means we are no longer sharing a common set of agreements about everything in the world and that ultimately, we the caregivers have lost control. Have you ever been to a fancy hotel and been caught off guard as the bellhop or doorman pauses waiting for a tip that you were not expecting because the protocol was unfamiliar to you? This can be very disconcerting, yet Alzheimer's patients and their families experience this kind of discomfort routinely.

Understanding our own dependencies and needs here and our discomfort in communicating with someone "from another planet," we prepare ourselves to offer a friend or family member with Alzheimer's special grace. Here is how:

First, from the beginning to the end of the process, we accept them, we forgive them for inconveniencing us, and we remember them as the whole person they have always been and will always be. Just as our cancer patients in Case 1 and Case 2 were in no way diminished as people by their disease, your friend is in no way diminished at their core by a diagnosis of Alzheimer's disease.

Secondly, we recognize that our response to the breakdown of normal left-brain speech and behavior in our friend is based on *our dependency on these functions* and fear of losing them and is not a judgment of our friend. We accept and understand that once we move beyond our own fear and uncertainty here that we have no need to judge or evaluate our friend's behavior. We have no wish to evaluate them or diminish them because of our own fear. Their wholeness as a person you love and support is not tied to their handicap in these common functions. They are now and will always be the whole person you remember before the onset of Alzheimer's disease regardless of their reaction to you or the world that has been influenced by its perception of the disease.

Finally, your presence in this current situation, as a friend, spouse, or caregiver, is one of a strong, loving ally not influenced by the turbulence of the moment or society's representation of Alzheimer's as a descent into hell. Your willingness to connect with your friend on many levels of consciousness, to take communication beyond conventional left-brain chatter using experiences and the Alzheimer's Cards, and to joyfully embrace and accept this stranger who is a friend "from another planet" changes the rules. Joy for your friend is tied to long moments whether in a shared reality or quiet acceptance of their reality.

Think of Alzheimer's disease as a life sentence to live in the present tense, to release all history and conscious memory of the past, and to drop all activities, pressures, and anxieties that were connected with a possible future you were working to achieve. There are no conflicts, no daily schedule at work, no monthly budget or bills to pay, no social obligations, or regrets about things done or not done. There are only long moments. Also, there is no future. Death and fear of death lose their meaning. Death is an abstract concept that we connect with many negatives associated with the end of our lives. Not so, for the Alzheimer's patient, living in the present. Now, think of yourself as the bearer of gifts to this life, in the moment, "on another planet." The gift of being in the present yourself, of always respecting the rules on Altzair and not trying to impose "Earth-rules," of listening, loving, and supporting without testing and the compulsion to fix things. Now, you have the idea.

HEAR MY VOICE

The Agreements

As my diagnosis of Alzheimer's disease is confirmed, my heart is filled with fear and uncertainty and a longing for a normal life with you that will no longer be possible.

While I am mentally healthy and experiencing the symptoms of early stage Alzheimer's disease, it is important to me that we make plans now for the choices you will be making later, when I am less capable. Unlike most diseases, such as cancer, heart disease, or intestinal problems, where the patient can interact with both family and physician throughout the course of the disease, Alzheimer's shuts down that communication quickly because the basis for it, a shared view of reality and healthy mental functioning, are no longer present.

Our agreements will be defined by a survey instrument in Appendix B called "My Alzheimer's Choice Book." This booklet expresses my wishes for how I would like to be treated at each stage of the disease process and how I would like you, my caregiver, to treat yourself.

I know that the statements I make now about how I wish to be treated in the future contain a great deal of uncertainty because neither of us really knows what the future will bring. So please use "My Alzheimer's Choice Book" as a rough guide, not a literal description of how to deal with future situations. I understand that no one can fully anticipate how Alzheimer's disease will impact them physically and mentally and that choices made in my current state of mind may not always apply to my circumstances at a later time. Regardless of this ambiguity, I am asking you to honor the spirit and details of the agreements in "My Alzheimer's Choice Book" whenever possible.

With Love and Great Appreciation for Your Service as My Caregiver.

_____

(Your signature)

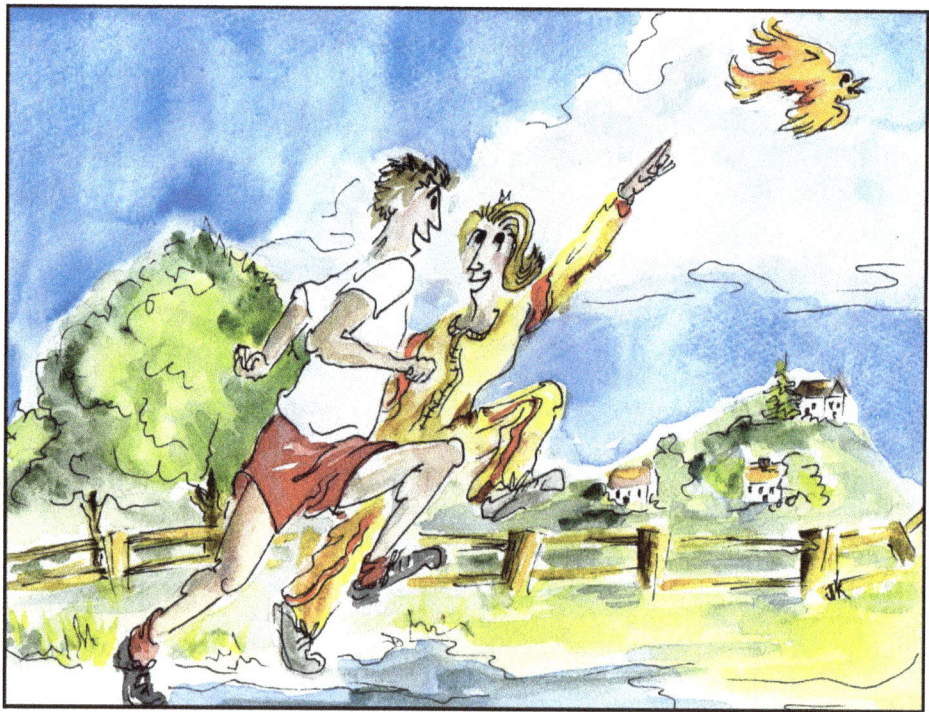

Good times ahead ... maybe.

Chapter 4: Tom and Jennifer

Jennifer: "I can feel you withdrawing, week by week, day by day, hour by hour, moment by moment.

"I know it's not your fault, but I find myself frustrated and angry with you. This was our time, my time. It seems that we've spent our whole life together waiting—waiting for the right job, waiting to have children, waiting for them to be in school and then finishing high school and college—waiting for you to retire, waiting to travel, waiting for our time together.

"It's not fair. I'm trapped here with you. I cannot let you out of my sight or you'll be undressing in the middle of the day, watching an empty TV screen, or wandering in our neighbor's back yard. You are like an infant. I love you, but it's not fair.

"Where are you? Why don't you answer my questions? Why can't I count on you? Why aren't you here for me? What is happening to us? Where are you?

"I feel so alone, so disconnected from our family and friends. Everyone is sympathetic but no one understands. Do you know how embarrassing it was last Sunday when you walked around introducing yourself to complete strangers? Or, when asked about your family, you said you didn't have one.

"I don't know what to do. I cannot care for you at home anymore. I'm exhausted, even with friends and family trying to relieve me. I cannot imagine you in a nursing home. What happens to my life?

"Why don't you try harder? I feel you slipping away. You're not trying to remember, to pay attention so we can enjoy our time together, to recognize the friends and family that visit. I know it's difficult but please try to be with us … *try*.

"I love you."

Tom: "I know you are frustrated. I can see it in the way you look at me. Embarrassed in one moment, angry in the next, then loving and concerned in the next.

"I am here for you right now but this may last for an hour or only a few minutes. What I don't have right now is control. Every moment is like walking along the edge of a cliff and never knowing when I will step off the trail into the abyss or when and how I can return.

"In your world, intentionality is very strong. If you will it to happen—to fix a meal, write a letter, have a conversation, dress, or any of a thousand other behaviors—chances are it will happen. Your intentions guide your behaviors. In my world, intentions are just like clouds that drift through a summer sky. At times I can hang on to an idea and stay focused; other times the cloud just drifts away and what I wanted or intended is lost.

When I was in high school in Gallatin, Tennessee, one of Mom's sisters, who had been close to us for many years, broke off communication with Mom based on a simple misunderstanding. Mom, one of the kindest people on the planet, reached out several times to try and make contact and was rebuffed. It was only later that she learned that the sister was suffering from dementia and very sensitive (to the point of being mildly paranoid) about any form of communication that suggested things were happening without her knowledge or being concealed from her. I think, in retrospect, it is likely that these were just the symptoms of progressing Alzheimer's disease, but at this point in time, old age, dementia, Alzheimer's disease, and mental illness were often confounded.

"I love you and want to please you. I want more than anything to have my life with you returned, to take the cruises we planned, to move to Colorado, to celebrate every evening with your company. I don't want to be helpless and needy and confused, but I no longer control what happens in my life. I feel so helpless.

"In this moment, I am in the world we have always shared, but my stay here is temporary. What I need is for you to join me, not be angry with me when I unintentionally cross the boundary to the planet Altzair, where I am no longer in control. If you are frustrated with me, imagine how frustrated I am with myself as my intentions no longer control my actions. Suddenly, I am the child or infant who has only a few limited ways to communicate my needs.

"What I live with every day now is fear, fear of the future, fear of the moment, and whether or not my mind will choose to be here or choose to be gone. I've had many diseases throughout my life and always before the diagnosis brought a special kind of relief. Knowing the cause of the illness meant that I could start the treatment and eventually expect a cure. With Alzheimer's disease, all I know is that today will be better than tomorrow, and a few years from now tomorrow will be much, much worse for me and for you, my loving caregiver.

"Hold me, love me, and in this long moment, remind me of whom we are and all that we share in this world."

* * *

In my experience with friends and family dealing with Alzheimer's disease, the conversation above is probably too articulate and packs too much information into just a few sentences. But it expresses the essence of the relationship between many partners when one is stricken with Alzheimer's disease.

Early stage Alzheimer's is often dominated by the emotions. The shock of a diagnosis that even though expected in many cases is still devastating. There's the frustration of not mastering the roles and tasks that are part of everyday life; the disappointment of giving up on a future that has been many years in the planning and may have a lifetime of work behind it; the fear, not just of dying, but of a well-proscribed path to death that is worse than ending life; the loss of independence in our shared world with a progressive dependence on a health care system that is filled with its own uncertainties about Alzheimer's and how to provide long-term care for Alzheimer's patients; and last, but definitely not least, there is the cost, the economic cost that is beyond the means of many families, the emotional cost for everyone involved, and finally the cost in personal time, health, and stress that often impacts the caregiver.

As you struggle with the negatives here in dealing with a family member or friend with early stage Alzheimer's, there are several important things to remember.

Acceptance. Denial and wishing things were different is very natural but not helpful because these actions block your path to health and happiness. When you accept what has happened, there is always hope and the opportunity for a life filled with many joyful moments. Is there hope that the Alzheimer's will suddenly go into remission? Not likely, any more than there is hope that a severed arm will suddenly grow back. But, there is always hope and there are always conversations you can have with yourself that move you toward hope instead of away from it. That is the choice you can make now and keep on making throughout the progression of Alzheimer's.

Several years ago, I lost my son Logan in a tragic accident. He died in my arms after an hour of CPR on a mountain top. The conversations I had with myself immediately after the accident were filled with anger and fear. Losing my son was the realization of my worst fear, one without realizing it I had rehearsed over and over. For a week I was lost in grief and confusion. As I began to emerge back into this world, a voice said to me, "You have a choice to make. You can choose to blame yourself, to say things to yourself about anger or mistakes or how your life is ruined in a way that can never be fixed, or you can say things that are healthy and constructive and send you on a path that, over time, will bring healing and joy back into your life." I was fortunate to make the right choice and my life has been blessed in many ways since. Now the choice is yours.

Mary was a sweet, quiet Italian woman with a big smile. She would reach out and grab my hand, pull me close, and gently tell me something that only she understood. Everyone loved Mary except Norma. For some reason, which only Norma knew, she didn't like Mary. If the aides put these two ladies side by side, Norma would hit Mary and yell obscenities at her. One day Mary arrived in the dining room with a new hairstyle ... her gray hair had been dyed a lovely shade of red. When Mary was seated next to Norma at the dining table, I waited for the fireworks to begin. But Norma just smiled at Mary, patted her hand, and carried on a babbled conversation. With Mary's new hair color she became Norma's new best friend!

What you say is what you get. As either the caregiver or the individual with a diagnosis of Alzheimer's disease, find the words to say to yourself that bring the most balance and happiness and joy to your life now, in this moment; then, do this, to the best of your ability for the rest of your life. If you have Alzheimer's, please understand that this kind of complex, directed self-talk, similar to an actual conversation, will be possible only in the early stages of the disease. Later, the sentences will be brief and will eventually become words or images or be lost completely, but the actions you take now, in the early stages, pave the way for the more limited communication to be meaningful. As the caregiver your words will change over time, but if you focus on acceptance, joy, and listening, there is nothing you can do that will provide more benefit to your friend or family member with Alzheimer's.

Why is this self-talk so important? We live in a world dominated by left-brain conversations and left-brain perceptions of our shared reality. Human consciousness is much more complex, and as Alzheimer's attacks and eventually ravages this part of our mind, other layers of consciousness will become progressively more important. To step away from our tendency to evaluate and suffer from negative ruminations and fears about your friend with Alzheimer's, you must start with your own self-talk.

What is self-talk? Self-talk is that running conversation that you have with yourself about everything, from the moment you get up until the moment you fall asleep. It guides you through your choice of clothes for the day, planning the day's schedule, what you focus on at work, what you worry about, how you relax and much, much more. It is actually very difficult for most people to "turn it off" and this frequently requires some special practice through meditation or other exercises. Self-talk has an enormous impact on shaping our personal view of reality. If we say negative, critical things to ourselves, our personality and our world tends to have a lot of negatives. If we are largely having positive self-talk conversations focused on healthy outcomes, then the chances are good that we will have a happy, fulfilled life. Think of self-talk as your personal radio with lots of options for stations that you can tune into to receive many kinds of messages.

When I described the self-talk process to students or clients, all immediately acknowledged that it is taking place in their minds. In fact it is very rare to find someone who does not "talk to themselves." Thinking about self-talk, however, immediately raises another question. If it is you and your mind that is talking, who is listening? Are there really two (or more) people in that space between your ears!

The quick answer, as I discussed in chapter 2, is that human consciousness is much like our personality, complex and multifaceted. You as an individual have many personalities or identities depending on what you are doing. You have an identity at work, another at home with your spouse, another with your children or friends, another under stress or on vacation. Your core personality underlies all of these situations but you may behave very differently in each because you have learned to tune your personality to the situation's specific requirements. Human consciousness is similar in that there are many forms of consciousness that operate together simultaneously even though you are not aware of this happening.

The talker and listener are simply two dimensions of your consciousness engaged in a very common process known as *self-referral.* Your talking part of the mind keeps up a continuous running dialog about what you are doing in the world now, what you did in the immediate past, and what you are going to do in the future.

This process is called *self-referencing* because, in this moment, you are referencing your past, present, and future to guide your actions. The listener plays an important role here because, like a good friend, he/she allows your thoughts to be heard, considered, and evaluated both logically and intuitively, referencing a full range of knowledge and memories.

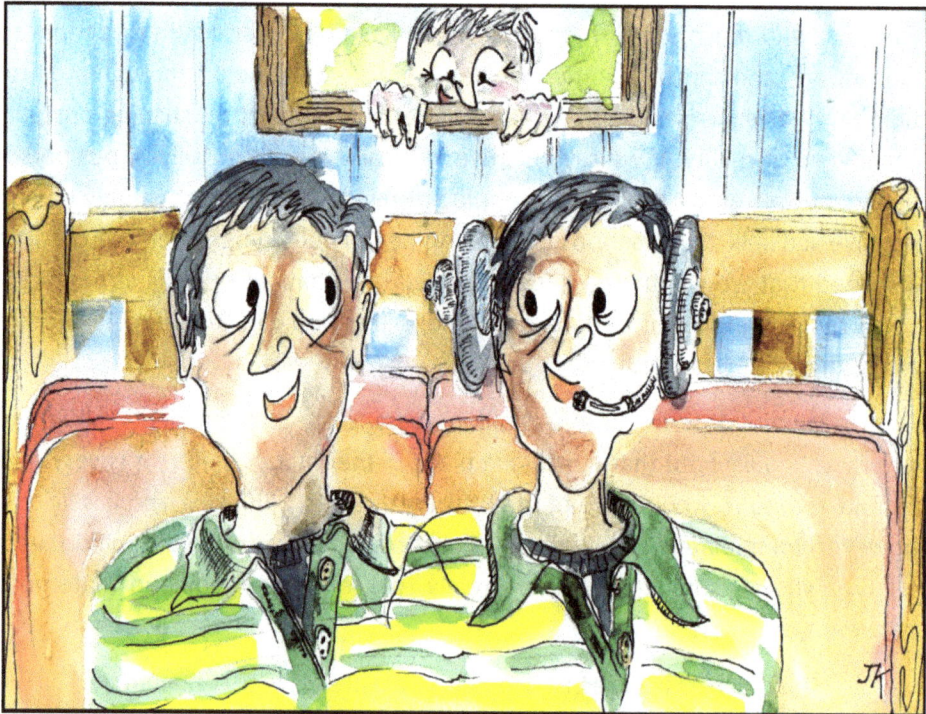

Say, your voice sounds very familiar to me...

The self-referencing part of self-talk is one of the early causalities in the progression of Alzheimer's disease because it is a recursive, cyclic process that requires a clear understanding of discrete stages in time and what is happening at each stage. Take the everyday behavior of "getting dressed" in the morning. As you are walking through the steps of showering, shaving, selecting clothes, and dressing, you are referencing many other things: the time (or how long you have to finish), what will happen later in the day (do you need to dress up, for example, for a special meeting), what your partner or spouse is doing (will you be coordinating a ride with them), what the weather is like, and so forth. As the ability to deal with a logical sequence of events in time that requires decision-making is diminished by Alzheimer's, self-talk becomes less reliable as a guide to making good choices because it is a left-brain function. This is why simple,

well-organized environments that help reinforce the correct choices are very helpful. They provide a sequence of clues that help keep the self-conversations focused and on track for everyday tasks.

Think of this problem in another way. Imagine that it is your friend or partner with Alzheimer's disease and that we have been able to replace the natural (and now limited) voice speaking in your friend's head with the voice of a robot. This is a very special robot, programmed to help reduce the symptoms of Alzheimer's. For example, the robot remembers the sequence of things to be done in the morning, from showering to getting dressed, and so always has the correct words available at the correct time. ("Now select a dress shirt from the closet and put it on.") When your friend gets off track, the voice steers them back onto the path with the best possible words. ("Stop for a moment. Put on your socks first; then it will be time

My son Logan and I battled from the moment he was born until shortly after his second birthday over who was in control—over eating, bathing, bedtime, and much more. I was the loser in most of these battles and probably would have kept on losing until my wife handed me a book called The Terrible 2's or something like that. Choices. He needed choices. From that moment on I stopped trying to control him and gave him choices. It became a game. He knew he was being manipulated but in a loving, caring way and started to enjoy the absurd options: "Would you rather go to bed now and have a story or have all of your fingernails pulled out?" Alzheimer's patients need clear choices also (with just two options), but they also need our humor, our willingness to be real with them as adults (try adding a dirty joke now and then to your conversation for spice), and unconditional acceptance of them and their condition.

to put on your shoes.") While this process will not be perfect, you would still see a significant improvement in your friend's behavior.

At the everyday level, with the exception of the times that you as the caregiver can be there to see that your partner is dressed and fed, there is no robot or constructive voice available. It is a nice idea but not realistic, and, with the self-referencing part of the mind damaged by Alzheimer's, management of everyday tasks will continue to deteriorate. At the emotional level, however, self-referencing is not so relevant, and even when it is present, the lack of a standard helps minimize the importance of the process. For example, how do you know you are sad or happy? Often these emotional states are defined by what you say to yourself. When you say to yourself you are happy, you are much more likely to be happy. That process has been demonstrated in hundreds of research studies. It is a simple tuning process: What you say to yourself has a strong influence on how you feel.

To manage the emotional dimensions of Alzheimer's disease, focused self-talk for both the caregiver and the patient becomes very important. A question I have often been asked about this type of positive self-talk is, "How can you ask me to lie to myself. If I don't believe I am well or happy or successful, how can telling me this possibly help?" The answer is as close as your heart. Your reality is not a fixed, rigid ice sculpture, alone on an arctic island, impervious to outside forces. Rather it is more like clay waiting to be molded by intentions. What is your choice here? To make the best of the current situation by flowing with it in a constructive manner or to make yourself miserable by feeding into all of its negative aspects?

Find words to care for yourself. As the caregiver, the first step you will need to take to help your friend with Alzheimer's is to tune your own mind to the right "station." Until your self-talk conversations are headed in the right direction, it will be difficult to deal with the fear and other emotions associated with Alzheimer's and provide the support your friend needs. The concept of an affirmation may be helpful here. An affirmation is simply a special kind of focused message that you say to yourself, with some repetition, to be sure you are sending your mind and your consciousness in the best directions for health, for inner peace, and for understanding and serving your friend. Think of an affirmation as a short, focused advertisement that you give to yourself to help tune your mind so that your self-talk is optimized.

Here are some examples of caregiver affirmations. They were created by Janet Edmunson for her clients serving as Alzheimer's caregivers.

* * *

Caregiver Affirmations
by Janet Edmunson, M.Ed.

I will hold on to my passions, because they are the essence of who I am.
I will give myself credit for staying strong despite being pushed to my limits.
I will give myself grace when I occasionally blow it.
It's perfectly normal to grieve even before my loved one dies.

I will explore life's adventures together.
I will look for the gifts that only this type of tragedy can afford.
I will let the love flow, even when all else is lost.
I will expect that some people will find it difficult to visit my loved one.
That's okay—it doesn't mean that they've stopped caring.

I will make it easier to get through difficult times by creating traditions to memorialize my loved one.
I will make meaning out of this disease.

* * *

Find words to guide your friend's self-talk. Equally important to affirmations for caregivers are the suggestions we give to Alzheimer's patients to guide their self-talk. While some cognitive functions, especially speech-related functions, are impaired by the disease, conversations remain an important channel of communication throughout all stages, even when the essence of the conversation may just be a few words or simple expression. A wealth of anecdotal information suggests that self-talk continues during the progression of the disease, but, as expected, it is less and less connected to a shared reality and more inner-oriented. Also, while self-talk in healthy individuals is often tied to activities and functions, self-talk in Alzheimer's patients is more likely to be tied to what they are experiencing on Altzair, such as dreams, memories, experiences, and feelings (in other words, words not strongly tied to Earth-reality). While self-talk will become more detached from our reality, Alzheimer's patients will however continue to be responsive to verbal or conversational input throughout the course of the disease. Obviously this communication becomes more limited over time and the response less predictable, but speech remains an important channel especially tied to basic functions such as bathing, dressing, dining, and visits by caregivers or doctors and therapists. An affirmation for someone with Alzheimer's becomes a simple, consistent message repeated daily or more often that impacts the mind with familiar, positive thoughts. Even with limited effectiveness for the individual with Alzheimer's, they are still important because a repetitive message will have a significant impact in a mind where thoughts are often fragmented or disorganized. There is also no doubt that in the earlier stages of the disease they are helpful in reducing stress and producing a more positive outlook.

What we say to ourselves shapes and defines much of our reality and so it is not surprising to find that this process continues even in individuals with Alzheimer's disease. The affirmation below was prepared by Barbara Derrick for her friend Wally. It was designed to be delivered as a recording to be used at bedtime. In my own work in health and sports helping people develop affirmation programs, I consistently found the combination of a relaxed or meditative state plus the affirmation was highly effective. When you create an affirmation that is more than a few words, remember that the Alzheimer's mind can quickly lose touch with the present and hence lose the meaning of the affirmation or the instructions to relax, so reminders of the purpose of the affirmation within the context of relaxation need to be present in almost every section.

* * *

Affirmations for Wally
by Barbara Derrick, Ph.D.

As you relax, you are experiencing quiet, peace, happiness, and joy. You can feel God's love surrounding you. This allows you to rest in the knowledge that God's love is guiding you, helping you in every way to make each day good and purposeful. You have good, appreciative feelings for those around you, knowing that you wish every person in your life well and they hold you in high regard.

Your mind will move toward functioning well, and this will give you great pleasure. Your short-term memory is improving, your mind more alert, and your recall of names and words improving day by day.

This time of relaxing will help to coordinate your nervous system and improve circulation through your body. The eliminating systems are removing toxins from your body. The foods that you eat will provide nourishment to your body.

You will be calm and cooperative to those around you at all times. You are self-sufficient. This makes you happy and proud. You will look forward to each day and enjoy life. Your short-term memory and your recollection of words and names are serving you well.

You are being healed—you are becoming whole at all levels. The divine energy within you is rejuvenating your body, mind, and spirit.

The planet Altzair is just on the horizon now. Your friend's visits to this new reality may be brief but there is little doubt those visits are happening. In the harsh light of this world, the subtle nuances of Altzair's mixture of dreams, shared memories, and sudden shifts in time or place can be terrifying, especially if judgment is involved. Remember the experience of an imaginary playmate (or perhaps a daydream) that was so real in your mind that the boundaries between this personal world and our shared world became unclear? Over time, society, through the process of social reinforcement, gradually conditioned you to live mostly full-time in the shared world, but still your dreams and other experiences that are not shared are very important.

Listen. Not sharing worlds is OK. What may have saved you as a child was the kindly mom or dad or friend who listened to your stories of an "imaginary" world or playmates and was wise enough to bless them with quiet understanding rather than shining a left-brain spotlight on them ("If we cannot both see it, then it is imaginary and doesn't really exist in this world. Grow up!"). That spotlight comes soon enough for most children as they enter kindergarten and then elementary school, where personal realities are often not tolerated. More and more your friend's visits to Altzair will be visits to a land of dreams and daydreams and memories that you cannot share. What you can share, however, is the emotions attached to them and the underlying anchors tied to your feelings and perceptions that operate in both worlds. Pain, hunger, confusion, joy, serenity, comfort, and a hundred other concepts represented by the Alzheimer's Cards remain meaningful in both worlds.

Think of your child coming home from a summer baseball game. You are sitting in the kitchen waiting as she walks in the door anticipating her reactions, winning or losing, where you will share in her joy or sadness, regardless. With Alzheimer's disease, you don't have to be present full-time to join in the flow of your friend's experiences and to share their emotions. As you will see in later chapters, there is a tendency to want to test a friend with Alzheimer's disease ("Do you remember Aunt Jessie and the trip we took to Chicago?"). Much of this testing can be very benign in everyday Earth-reality, but realize what it represents. This is really your attempt to force the conversation back into your familiar, shared world, where you live every day and are most comfortable. This is a world where evaluation is a natural part of most communication. Testing to see how much your friend will remember, and the assumption that this remembering, if successful, is somehow important as proof they are still sharing *your* world is very stressful and unfair.

Relax. Enjoy the presence of your friend. Watch for their emotions and look for opportunities to bring peace and joy by joining them here rather than fishing in their world and then, when you get a bite, rushing to pull this shared memory to the surface. Go with the flow.

* * *

Tom: "How you can help me most now.

"It sounds trite but both of us will live until we die. I may die sooner and when I die there is a good chance I will not remember you or be part of your world. But until that time we have hundreds of moments together. All I ask is that you join me in those moments without fear and without reservation. Neither of us would call our life hopeless because we are going to eventually die, so my life with Alzheimer's is not hopeless. It's different. It is not the path I would choose, if I had a choice, but it's the road that I am traveling. I hate missing many of our shared dreams and plans. I hate it that I will be dependent on you in ways that we had not planned.

"What I want from you is that when you think about me embrace all parts of me, the parts we share and the parts while I am dreaming. As you talk to yourself about me, turn loose any negative feelings and just accept in this moment who and what I am without evaluating it. When your mind is clear and you can be with me without conflict that is a gift that is precious beyond imagination. As time passes I will become a stranger to you, a person you do not know who in turn does not remember you. Please accept and love that stranger as you love and accept me now. That stranger is an alien only in this artificial world we have created in our minds. In my heart and body, at the soul of my being, I will always be the person you have known and will always remember you even though we no longer share the same world.

"When I would daydream in the past, you would tease me about being on another planet. Well, at the moment, I am on another planet, one where you typically cannot join me with words and shared thoughts. But there is still time for you to be with me in many other ways. My consciousness now is divided into moments that grow shorter and shorter every day, but in those moments I am here with you, comforted by your presence. Whether I am on the Earth or Altzair no longer matters. All I need is for you to be present with me."

HEAR MY VOICE

The Environment

We have both noticed that my symptoms are getting worse and that both short-term memory and my ability to perform everyday tasks such as dressing or preparing a meal are deteriorating. More and more you want to make decisions for me and to protect me, which I appreciate. You are also starting to see the first signs of the "stranger" that I will eventually become.

My mind and voice are still very strong though and wherever possible there are still many choices I would like to make. I am still strongly connected with your Earth-reality. Please accept that when I make a choice, a few minutes later I may not remember that choice and change my mind or be frustrated by the choice or have some other reaction that suggests the choice was wrong. This is not the case. In the long moments we have together, the choices I am making are real choices and important to me.

I can think about and often want to have a voice in most daily decisions—what I am wearing, where we might go during the day, what foods are appropriate, what to watch on TV, what to do in our home or wherever we may be.

How can you help me make these choices? Since you cannot be with me every moment (and neither of us would want this anyway), you can help to make the choices easier for me to understand by creating an environment that is structured to help me remember how to function every day when I forget. The movie *Fifty First Dates* is the story of my life now. Every morning not only starts a new day for me, in many respects it is a new life where the tasks, the people, the environment, and everything else are a mixture of the familiar and the new.

Please look at the recommendations for improving my living environment in chapter 7 and use your best judgment here to make them work for me.

Thank you for your love and support!

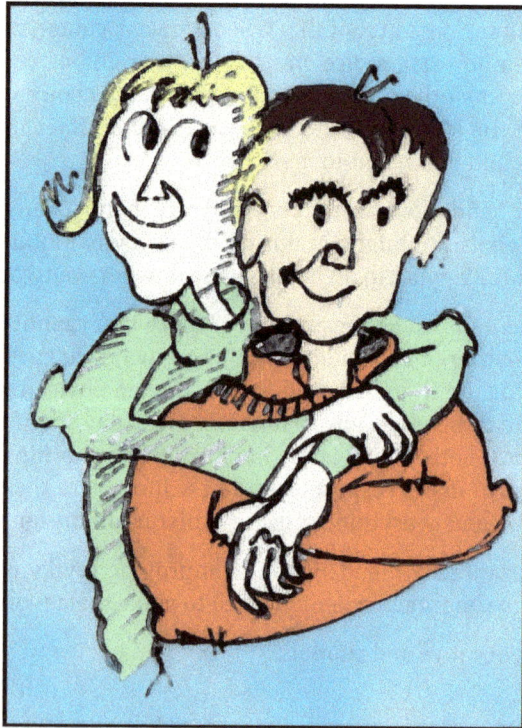

I love you unconditionally now and forever.

Chapter 5: Love, Flow, and Time

The progression of Alzheimer's is about a journey to death that is as certain as taxes and other facts that anchor our physical and social realities. As you can see from Tom's last comments, there are many ways you can choose to deal with this trip ... you can fight it, you can ignore or deny it, or you can embrace it much the same way you would embrace the outcome of any life event.

When we think about Tom and Jennifer or the other couples, families, and friends we will encounter in later chapters, we are largely thinking about love because it is love that binds the patient and caregiver throughout the progression of the disease. It matters little whether the love is physical, passionate, and romantic or just friendly. Love will be different now, and throughout the book we will touch on the meaning of love. The biggest change for you here will be around what love does *not* mean. On the Earth love is a shared consensual experience, perhaps a candlelight dinner, a conversation, a concert, lovemaking, and a host of other things. On Altzair these rules are different already and will change more as time passes.

Love based on shared moments in this world will become less and less frequent over time and more and more one-directional as you look for examples of events or memories you can share while acknowledging that these experiences are becoming less and less important and accessible to your partner. Love based on warmth, kindness, touch, listening, and other factors that I will discuss in later chapters will, to a degree, always be needed and can often be reciprocated by your partner. Of course you know the common stereotype, which is that in the later stages of Alzheimer's disease your partner will not recognize you, and this is very likely to be true. However, this stereotype is largely based on our shared, left-brain world where one of the most common, consensual understandings is that we know each other's name and can communicate it. Throw that idea out the window and replace it with just the simple concept of "familiarity" and you open up whole new landscapes where love and other kinds of shared moments can exist. My Aunt Emilou, to whom this book is dedicated, is one hundred and has been in late stage Alzheimer's for the past six years, but several times a week she and her daughter Katherine find a familiar place to share, even when both are on different planets! More about this later.

Another key kind of love that is especially important in the early stages of Alzheimer's is unconditional acceptance. This is the heart of what was described in the previous chapter when I mentioned several examples of self-talk and suggest that it avoid evaluation as much as possible. This is difficult to do because much of the daily clutter in our mind is about evaluation. How do you look this morning? How was the cup of coffee or breakfast? Did you make it to work on time? What is the latest office gossip? The boss didn't like the report you submitted ... why? You get the point. Typically a large percent of self-talk concerns evaluations or judgments about almost everything around you, and it is difficult for this not to carry over to your partner with Alzheimer's. Yet, you also know intuitively that unless you are addressing a life-threatening situation that needs your action immediately, the evaluations and the running stream of self-talk feeding these evaluations is not helping.

> My golfing friend Ted was only sixty when the first signs of Alzheimer's disease appeared. On the golf course there was no sign of a problem. We had so many side bets going in our foursome that losing track of the score, as he was prone to do, was not unusual. It was over drinks at a club dinner that his wife Gail first informed us of his diagnosis. The early symptoms were very mild. There were examples of forgetting and losing track of things, but it was Tom's behavior in the morning that concerned Gail. He would wake early, have a cup of coffee, which was brewed automatically, and then on some days just get stuck. Gail would wake an hour later and find him sitting at this desk, not sure what he was doing there or that he had a schedule for the day to keep. Soon after the dinner, he and Gail moved to Cincinnati to be with family.

Unconditional acceptance means you watch, you listen, you laugh, you cry, you empathize, and for the most part, you simply let things be. You stay away from the left brain's tendency to want to control everything. You can control few things in your friend's life now, especially things that relate to their thinking and behavior, and trying will simply frustrate you both. Acceptance and the love that stems from it say clearly that you are present but not in control, at least not in the typical logical/verbal left-brain kind of control we are all familiar with.

Another dimension of love ties very closely to time, both physical, or "clock," time and personal, or psychological, time. In our shared consensual reality, much of this sharing is tied to time. You have an urgent need to call your boss, finish this visit, smoke a cigarette, or whatever. I respect that. It is part of the unwritten rules of our world. You need to deal with an urgent matter? Fine,

58

go ahead, I understand. On Altzair, however, a whole different set of rules is in place for time. There can still be urgency but this is not the norm. What is quickly lost here is the consensus about what time means. This understanding is unlikely to cross the boundary between your friend's world and your world. In your world there are things to do and after visiting with your friend there is another appointment or activity probably already on your calendar. As a result, when you try to hurry up things based on this agenda, you are very likely to create a tear or discontinuity in your partner's world and add a dose of anxiety for good measure. They are in the present. There is no set of future activities or deadlines pending in their mind. They will not understand your schedule and deadlines. But on some level, they will sense your impatience, which will make them anxious and may destroy the quality of the moment.

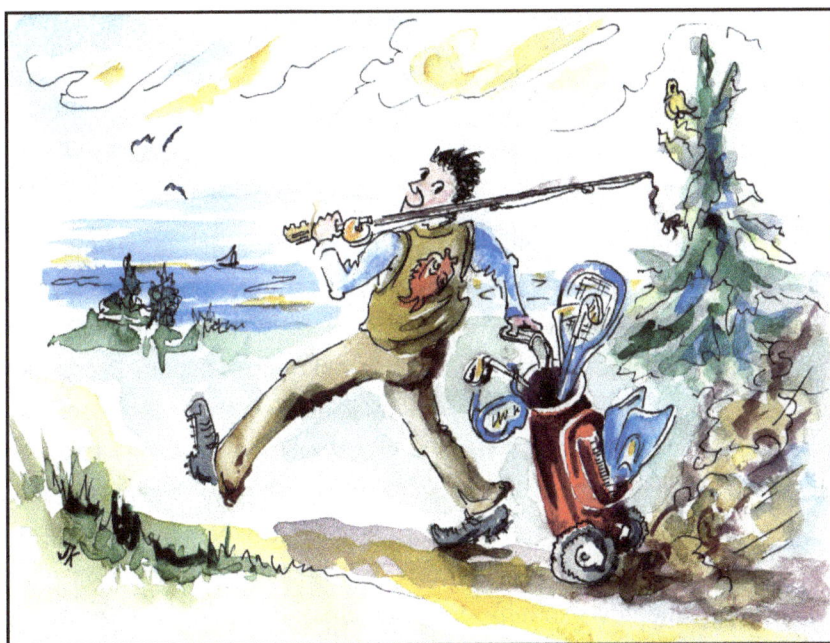

Living joyfully, effortlessly in flow

Flow is one of my favorite terms from sport psychology. An athlete is "flowing" when their performance is effortless and natural versus forced, as if they have to expend effort and thought to perform. I am sure you also under-stand flow in relationships and can think of many situations where you and a friend or partner were so much in tune with each other that words were largely superfluous. Unconditional acceptance of your friend with Alzheimer's is really about flow. You are present. You are listening. Your mind is largely quiet so that when the opportunity to just be with this friend without judgment occurs, you can interact with them in flow, allowing whatever wants to happen, happen without feeling the need to force it or control it. You become an interested observer, not the driver in this case.

Time in our shared world on Earth is not the same as time on Altzair. Our behavior in virtually every setting on Earth is tied to the clock. It defines when we awaken in the morning, when we go to school or work or play, when we dine, and the "when" associated with most other events during the day. The "when" dimension of our day carries with it a certain amount of tension or pressure to comply because in a shared reality where, by consensus, we agree on the rules, time underlies almost every agreement. You will be "at this place" or "involved in this activity" or "with this person" at specific times. And, no, you cannot take this for granted without crossing a number of social boundaries that have significant consequences. Wearing a watch is a common way of continually keeping track of the time dimension. Calendars and schedules add structure to this dimension, reinforcing its importance as an agreement between us about how we will share and conduct our lives.

In addition to the "when" dimension of time, which drives most of our behaviors during the day, there is an equally important "how long" dimension to this component of our shared reality. How long will you spend at lunch or driving to work or in a conversation with a friend over cocktails? Every event in time carries with it a "how long" expectation and, if there is a conflict with someone over time (unless you have a friend who is habitually late), this is where the conflict will occur. One of you expects more or less of a time commitment for the meeting you are having, or perhaps there is a deadline that suggests that within a certain time you will have accomplished specific goals, or finally, perhaps time flows so differently for you and your colleagues that sharing is difficult—you are on urgent, "get-it-done" time and they are on Maniana time.

When this happens, because we all tend to be constantly evaluating ourselves and others, you are evaluating yourself or being evaluated by others. Right? And, a miss here can be very stressful.

Go back to Jennifer's frustration with Tom and his struggles with everyday tasks. Tom's world gets out of synch with the world he and Jennifer have shared for many years when he has trouble dressing or forgets to dress before he goes outside. Jennifer is frustrated. *Why are you acting like a baby? Please get dressed.* Tom is frustrated. *What is the rush. My mind has wandered somewhere else.* The result is a conflict that looks like a conflict over behavior when the real issue is time. In linear, everyday Earth-time, there are long established expectations about what will happen during the day at certain times and how long this will take. During the course of Alzheimer's, the agreement to honor these expectations will begin to fracture, first in occasional moments such as the above example and then eventually vanish all together. There will be no agreements about time because linear, structured, task-oriented time simply does not exist on Altzair.

The dimension of time is so fundamental to all of our shared agreements in this world that it becomes the default for demonstrating that we share the same world. You and your partner both went out into the world independently and worked, played, shopped, or filled any other roles, then, at the agreed-upon time, you reconnected for dinner, an evening at home, or to simply go to bed together to sleep. Both of you honored the rules about time that we consensually accept in this culture. If you were running late, you called. If expectations on your to-do list needed to be met, you tried to accomplish them. Our cultural definition of communication for both work and play is tied to these understandings about time. Now things are changing. The clock on Altzair is not running at the same speed. Einstein's laws of relativity theory no longer apply. While it is focused on the present tense, time on Altzair can go forward and be similar to Earth-time, but, it can also go backward or sideways or even stop! To an observer on Earth, this can be frustrating and incomprehensible, but, to your partner on Altzair, it will make perfect sense.

Research on how people keep track of time adds to our understanding here. In experiments where subjects are prevented from seeing a watch or clock and asked to estimate the actual time under a variety of conditions, the results are very consistent. Most people carry a clock in their minds that is quite precise and their estimates of actual time on the clock are fairly accurate. When asked to estimate the time required to do certain tasks, such as reading a page of text or walking the length of a football field, they are still accurate. Finally, when asked to measure the time that has passed after some event (such as a person entering the room) and the present, these estimates are very close to the actual time. In other words, we not only share an external clock keeping track of time day and night, we have an internal clock that also keeps track. This internal sense of time as well as our ability to execute tasks that require a sequence of steps in time are both early casualties in the progression of Alzheimer's disease. Loving your partner on their journey, especially in the early stages of Alzheimer's, often requires taking a big step toward their world. Practically, this means that you quit expecting them to live in your linear time and follow the shared rules about Earth-time that you shared for so many years. Their internal clock is no longer tuned to the same time as yours. It also means that in order to enjoy the many long moments remaining, you take the pressure off of the "when" and "how long" experiences you will have with them at home and later in institutional settings and learn to simply be with them, there in that moment. If you can do this with humor and openness about your partner's changing world, so much the better. I am pretty dingy most of the time, so it is easy to laugh about that dinginess with my spouse or friends. Humor or gallows humor can change many disheartening situations into occasions for laughter during the course of Alzheimer's disease. That may be possible for you too. I have also learned that acknowledging your partner's journey and the disconnection from this world using the language of dreams or another planet can help. There is no joy in an Alzheimer's diagnosis, but that being said, it is what life is about for you and your partner or family member in the short term. There is a beauty and comfort in the frankness and transparency of discussions about any problem or condition. When my son died, most people were afraid to mention anything about him when actually I was hungry for people to ask. Most individuals with a disability want your real engagement with them that includes questions about the disability, not conversations that are superficial and designed to treat them as if their handicap didn't exist. If there is an elephant in the room, take note—it doesn't like to be ignored.

The same is true for individuals with Alzheimer's disease. They are hungry for acceptance of their reality. Gallows humor: they love it. Dirty jokes: bring them on. Your mistakes and foolishness: perfect. There is an adult there, caught in a trap that makes them appear at times unintelligent or childlike or lacking awareness. Ignore that and embrace the adult part of their minds with all of the irreverence and frankness and R-graded reality that you can muster.

Your assignment, if you choose to accept it, is to say the words needed in your own self-talk to allow you to accept your partner's condition without fear and also to provide the love needed for your partner to learn to accept and live in Altzair-time when you are with them, finding as much peace and joy as possible in every moment. Be in the present tense. Make your interactions about things that are concrete, not abstract, especially in the later stages of Alzheimer's. "What do you want for lunch?" is actually quite a challenging proposition compared to looking at several pictures of sandwiches and selecting the "ham sandwich." Limit the number of options in most cases to make the choices clear. From now on, you are their rock. You are the fountain that covers frustration and fear and the growing gaps in shared understanding between this world and their world with the warm waters of kindness and acceptance and the assurance that in whatever forms are appropriate, you will be there, in the present, with love.

HEAR MY VOICE

Could You Just Listen?

When I ask you to listen to me
and you start giving me advice,
you have not done what I asked.
When I ask you to listen to me
and you begin to tell me why I shouldn't feel
that way, you are trampling on my feelings.
When I ask you to listen to me and you feel you
have to do something to solve my problem, you
have failed me, strange as that may seem.
Listen! All I asked was that you listen,
not talk to or do—just hear me.
Advice is cheap; twenty cents will get you both
Dear Abby and Billy Graham in the same paper.
I can do for myself; I'm not helpless—maybe
discouraged and faltering, but not helpless.
When you do something for me that I can
and need to do for myself, you contribute
to my fear and inadequacy.
But when you accept as a simple fact that
I do feel what I feel, no matter how traditional,
then I can quit trying to convince you and
can get about this business of understanding
what's behind this irrational feeling.
When that's clear, the answers are obvious
and I don't need advice.
Irrational feelings make more sense
when we understand what is behind them.
Perhaps that's why prayer works, sometimes, for
some people—because God is mute and He/She
doesn't give advice to fix things. "They" just
listen and let you work it out for yourself.
So please listen and just hear me. And if you
want to talk, wait a minute for your turn—and
I'll listen to you.

—Anonymous

64

Chapter 6: Patrick and Julie

Patrick and Julie are sitting outside on a shaded porch with Alice Jackson, an administrator from the South Beach Extended Care Facility, when an elderly lady with a big smile on her face is pushed by in her wheelchair by a nurse's aide and parked in the sun.

Patrick: "She looks happy. Has she been here long?"

Alice: "Yes, for three years now. That is Emilou."

Patrick: "She looks pretty fit. Is she here in one of the elder care programs?"

Alice: "No she is in late stage Alzheimer's. She's doing well today, but she is one-hundred and her health is more up and down than is apparent. She's a very nice lady and has a wonderful daughter."

A nurse approaches and interrupts Alice briefly with a form to be signed. Alice turns back to Patrick and Julie noting that they are both more uncomfortable than on their last visit to explore the facility and discuss treatment options. Patrick looks exhausted.

"How are the two of you doing?"

Patrick looks at Julie and then says, "Not so well. It's been a tough week for both of us. Julie was fixing lunch last week while I was at work and cut herself, then had trouble stopping the bleeding and couldn't remember how to contact me. She ended up outside, in her nightgown, and was finally rescued by a neighbor, who kept things under control until I arrived. It was pretty scary. Julie does pretty well at home most of the time, but I'm almost afraid to leave her now."

Julie nods and then looks directly at Alice.

"I was scared and didn't know what to do. I couldn't remember how to call Patrick."

"And when I arrived at the apartment, I could see Julie was upset. I told her that she should never use the kitchen knife. It's too dangerous. This just made her angry. She said, 'You are a jerk. I needed help. Where have you been?' And I am giving you the PG version."

Julie grimaces and nods her head.

"I know. I'm so sorry. But you were so condescending. I hated it when you scolded me like I was a child."

She turns to Alice.

"I feel like a monster at times. Patrick will be trying to help and I will tell him to bug out, leave me alone, or call him a 'jerk' or much worse. What is happening here? Frustration? I hate to be treated like a child."

Alice turns toward Patrick.

"Is that true Patrick? How were you addressing Julie? In a tone that suggested she was a child?"

Patrick thinks for a second. "Well maybe. When Julie is upset, I guess that I do try to keep things simple and clear, possibly like I was explaining things to a child."

Alice pauses for a second, thinking, then leans back in her chair.

"I see several things happening here. First, being blunt or direct is just a part of the disease process, Julie. Part of the consensual reality that we share is an understanding about social interactions, especially with friends and loved ones. Most of the time, we tone down harsh, confrontational comments as a part of getting along with each other. That is not the norm, however, on Altzair, especially when you are frustrated. Many of the outlets for frustration such as wit or humor or even a defensive response are no longer available to Julie."

Patrick: "So you are saying that I can expect more of this?"

> *Visiting Aunt Emilou at her nursing home in Florida, it is obvious that she is very well cared for in an attractive, professional facility within an Alzheimer's unit. She doesn't recognize me, but is familiar with Katherine, her daughter, as a new friend. She is traveling in her past during our visit as a child and young adult, with her mother, and is clearly spending most of her time on the planet Altzair.*
>
> *While this sounds benign, it is not. Katherine's family has spent most of their retirement savings caring for Emilou the past five years. It would break Emilou's heart to know that while she lives in relative luxury, her family is having to sacrifice and that in the future, if they have severe dementia, the same opportunities for high-quality care will most likely not be affordable for them.*
>
> *Is there a line here that has been crossed? And if so, when do you know it is time to stop—and if you did know, could you make this decision?*

"Absolutely. Honoring conventional social agreements will be less and less important to Julie. She is trying to survive now in a world that doesn't always make sense, and blunt, direct communication may be the only way she can communicate with words."

"However, as I listen to the two of you, I am also thinking that you fed into this situation in a way Patrick that increased Julie's frustration leading to the angry response."

"How do you mean?"

"Imagine for a moment that I started to speak to you now as if you were a child, and in that tone of voice, I criticized you (Alice shifts her voice to that of a parent) perhaps because you put on different color socks this morning. You are wearing one black sock and one that is blue. That is pretty careless. Did you do that deliberately?"

Patrick frowns and makes a grumpy response.

"No. But that is not the same thing. I'm not a child. Neither is Julie, but she is acting like a child and so I want to be sure she understands me."

Alice: "No Patrick, Julie is not acting childlike. She is acting like an adult with Alzheimer's disease. There is a big difference. Even if she is confused at times, she is still an adult and will remain an adult throughout the course of the disease. When you speak to her as a child, her emotional reaction inside is just like your reaction a moment ago. She doesn't like it. She is an adult and it is very rude and condescending to treat her like a child."

"I'm sorry Julie."

"I know you are. It's OK."

Alice continues, looking directly at Patrick.

"And then you unknowingly added salt to the wound. You scolded or admonished her for using the knife! Once again that is a thing you would normally do with a child, not an adult. With an adult you would take a different approach. No wonder she is frustrated and angry.

"Alzheimer's disease cuts through the polite veneer of typical social interactions fairly quickly. More and more, if Julie has something to say, it will be direct! This is probably not intended as confrontational, but in an environment where conversations tend to be polite and indirect it may be perceived in that manner. Complex speech filled with innuendos and several levels of meaning is a nightmare for a person with Alzheimer's, so it is equally important for your speech to be direct also."

Julie turns to Patrick and starts to speak but pauses, looks at him momentarily, and then closes her eyes for a few moments.

"Please help me. I love you and I want to be with you but I'm so afraid. One moment I am in our lovely house and the next it is completely unfamiliar to me. I know I am embarrassing you but I cannot stop.

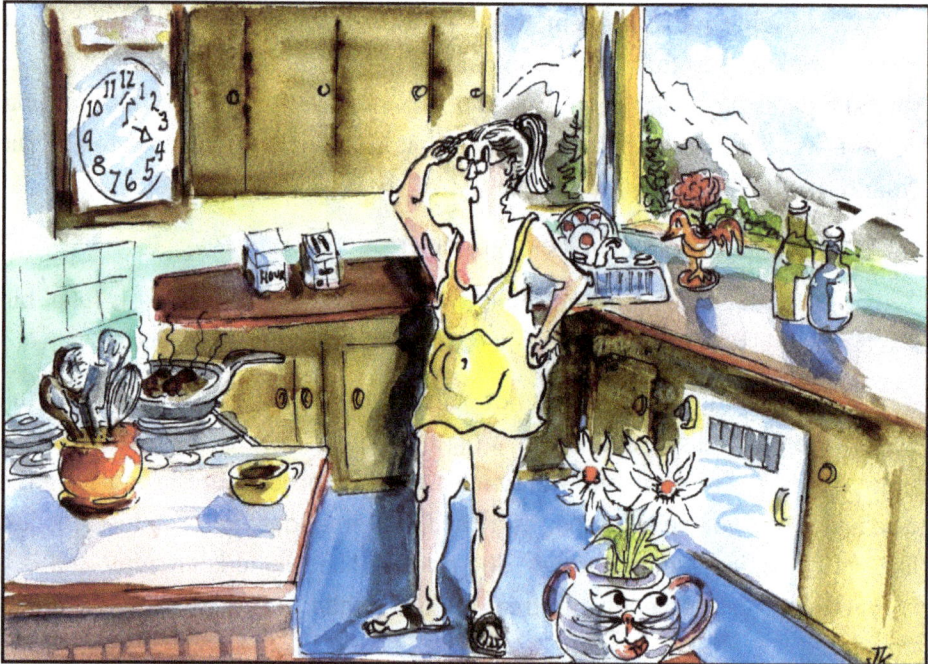

Let me see... is it time for breakfast or bed?

"I am having that awake-dream again. I'm in the kitchen. I know I belong there. Everything is familiar, the stove, the sink, the table with flowers that I love ... but I don't know why I am here. I see the bread on the table and the roast beef with the knife. Am I making a sandwich? I know how to do that? Is that why I am here?

"I love this nightgown. It's so cool and comfortable. But, it's the middle of the day. Why am I wearing this nightgown now? Am I going to bed or did I just get up? I don't remember. I think I would like to go outside into the sun. Where is Patrick? Am I awake or in a dream?"

Patrick watches Julie, then, after a moment, rests his hand on hers, inhales deeply, and turns to Alice.

"We are wondering what steps to take to give Julie the care she needs. My work as an attorney is not something I can do at home and we need the income. Is it time to hire a nurse to be there during the day? Or, is it time to consider your outpatient care program? That's what we are here to discuss.

"Unfortunately it looks like our insurance only provides coverage for residential programs and neither Julie nor I are willing to give up living together."

"No we are not! I don't want to live away from Patrick."

Alice: "As you can see, the time is coming when you will need full-time help with Julie, and Julie, you will want that help because if you don't have it, many precious moments with Patrick will be lost. The transition from early to middle stage Alzheimer's is extremely stressful for a caregiver, especially a spouse. Our experience here plus much evidence from research shows that Patrick will need to pay attention to caring for himself, in order to be able to support you adequately, and Alzheimer's caregivers are notorious about *not* giving themselves adequate care."

> *While visiting my mom in the nursing home, I often spend time observing other residents and their families. Mrs. Law has advanced Alzheimer's and doesn't speak, sucks her thumb, chews on her clothes, and has no interaction with her family. Her daughter visits often and we talk briefly while caring for our moms.*
>
> *One Sunday afternoon while approaching the dining room, I heard someone playing the piano. I was astounded when I walked in the room and saw Mrs. Law sitting at the piano and playing remarkably well. It was amazing to me to watch her play chords and recognizable tunes like "Moon River" while still in her demented state of mind.*

Patrick: "I feel so helpless. One moment Julie and I are a couple enjoying life together as we have for so many years; then, in a blink, she will be distracted and pulled into a different reality. Last Sunday, in church, we chatted with friends like old times. Then, near the end of the service, she suddenly stood up, looked and me, and said, "I don't belong here." The next thing I know, she is walking down the aisle, out the door to the street, looking for her ride. It was very embarrassing. I was able to get her back inside, and we watched the end of the service, standing in the aisle behind the last pew. Afterwards, our friends and the minister came to visit and offer words of comfort, but Julie didn't recognize them this time and grew more and more agitated. She didn't calm down until later, after we returned home."

Julie: "I remember being overwhelmed. The closeness of everyone at the church. I didn't understand why I was there. You looked like my husband, but I knew you were not my husband, yet, you had your arm around me. People were moving along the columns by the windows. Almost like shadows. I couldn't see them clearly. I had to get outside. Later, I was surrounded by people who seemed to know something about me that I didn't know. Why were those people wanting to be close to me and to touch or hug me? That was very uncomfortable."

Left-Brain Reality and Cause-Effect Sequences

One of the strongest attributes of our shared left-brain reality is the underlying logic of how things work in the real world. We often use the term *cause-effect* to describe this linear sequence of things in time. For example, "It is cold in here. I am going to walk across the room and close the window. Then I am going to light a fire." Or, perhaps, "It is lunchtime. I am going to get dressed and walk into the kitchen to fix a sandwich with the roast beef from last night; then, I am going outside on the porch to eat it." These simple actions are more than just routine tasks for the person involved: They are actually implied agreements that we make with each other because they represent the fundamental daily habits and routines that are the basis for our shared, consensual Earth-reality. In the above case, your actions to address the problem of discovering that the room is cold are likely to be very similar to my actions. We both will close the window and turn on the heat. The same is true for making a sandwich.

Alzheimer's disease, even in the early stages, can quickly begin to erode some of these agreements. If the behavior required of you is logical and linear—getting from Point A to Point B and then remembering why you wanted to be at Point B—then you cannot assume as the caregiver that you and your friend will be on the same wavelength here. As I discussed in chapter 2, Altzair time is not linear time, and so, communication between you and your partner based on linear time is going to break down at some point. What used to be a shared agreement about simple tasks such as "getting dressed" is no longer an agreement or an understanding between you. The more linear or sequential the task and the more steps along the way where there are decision points then the less you can rely on the existence of a clear path on Altzair to demonstrate this behavior and the greater the chance for confusion or frustration.

Complicating this process is the fact that the normal self-talk that would guide your partner through these steps is missing or distorted. While the self-talk program that suggests you "put on your socks and then put on your shoes" is still working in your reality, this simple, implied agreement or understanding may not be valid for your partner.

How then can you communicate if these everyday agreements are no longer valid? Imagine for a moment what it would be like to entertain someone from another country and a very different culture. Would you expect them to understand our table manners, how to make coffee with your state-of-the-art coffeemaker, how to operate the TV remote control, or many other behaviors that we take for granted? Probably not. The cause-effect agreements that are in place in our culture take some time to learn, and, to start with, you probably would not assume they were understood by this non-native visitor.

All similar assumptions are now off the table with your partner. You cannot count on our familiar logical agreements to serve as the basis for most communication any longer. In fact, as you will see below, by expecting these agreements to be in place, you will unfairly hinder your relationship and side-track the opportunity for long moments. Such agreements, for the most part, have little meaning on Altzair. However, in their place there is a whole universe of memories that you can count on because, for many years, they are likely to exist both in our shared Earth-reality and on Altzair. Three of the most important groups of memories you can share between worlds are sensory memories, some memories of life experiences, and certain physical or kinesthetic memories.* These memories are likely to remain intact when left-brain memories can no longer be called upon.

Experiences in the moment of sensory events such as sounds, sights, tastes, touch, and body sensations such as warmth open the door for shared communication that will persist throughout the course of Alzheimer's disease. You can be on the Earth while your friend or partner is on Altzair and find that conversation about the taste of food, the warmth of the sun, or the sound of the train whistle in the distance all have relevance and contribute to meaningful communication between you. The key here for successful communication is to remember that whatever you are discussing is in the present, not a bridge to connect back to the past. Let me give you an example.

One day let's assume that you decide to bring an old recording of your favorite dance songs from around the time you and your spouse were married. Included is a special favorite used for the wedding dance. With joy and good intentions in your heart, you play this for your spouse. For a moment, she is happy as she remembers the music, but her expression turns to a puzzled look and then quickly to one of frustration. She is in tears by the time you finish the tape. What has happened here?

Without intending it, you have tested her. She recognized quickly that this was a familiar piece of music. Her memory of experiences and the emotions connected with these experiences recognized this piece of music and that it was very significant, but her conscious mind, in the present with you, doesn't recognize it because it cannot connect back to her experiences with the music.

What she can understand, however, is that the music is familiar and you are expecting her to remember it, and when she cannot, it is very frustrating. In other words, with the best of intentions, you inadvertently set her up to fail. But had you brought other recordings that were not necessarily familiar to her, you could have enjoyed them together in the moment. What a joy to listen to music with someone you love.

Often kinesthetic memories that connect many of the sensory elements combined above provide even stronger anchors for sharing. These include walking, running, riding a bike, swinging a golf club, swimming, giving birth, and driving a car. Most of these are fair game for communication in both worlds. Often,

> *A very sweet lady named Matilda is in a wheelchair but her mind seems fine. She seems to crave conversation and I try to visit with her every time I visit Mom. She has told me she was a school teacher, has three daughters, and many grandchildren. As many times I have been in the nursing home, I have never seen anyone visiting Matilda.*
>
> *One day when she seemed particularly in need of company, I sat with her a while. She told me she had quit her job as a teacher to care for her mother. After moving her mother into her home, she gave her round-the-clock care until her passing. Her regret was that her mother passed away while Matilda was napping in another room. She felt guilty about that. I assured her that her Mom wanted it that way.*
>
> *My thoughts often go back to that conversation and feel sad that Matilda's daughters never visit their mom.*

in the moment you can enrich them with specific experiential memories as long as the cause-effect dimension is automatic. Driving to the beach with your family, giving birth to a daughter, playing golf at Hilton Head, these all offer important opportunities to share.

Notice that in both of these examples we are talking about a holistic or right-brain kind of experience that has more to do with a moment in time and the feelings associated with that moment than with a sequence of events in time. As you know, the sequence with its logical steps and the recursive properties that we depend on in our shared reality will be very challenging for your partner and may not be accessible. Recursion here refers to the fact that at each step in the sequence the person can "look back" to help understand why they are at this place. I have gone from the bedroom to the kitchen but in the kitchen forget why I am there. In Earth-reality it is easy for me to look backwards in the sequence to remember that I went into the kitchen to fix lunch. As Alzheimer's progresses, moving either way in a linear time sequence becomes more and more challenging.

* * *

Alice: "That process you are describing Julie, of feeling off-balance and uncertain about why you are in a certain place or doing a certain task, while not pleasant, is a normal part of Alzheimer's. In our shared world when your mind is healthy, everything is compartmentalized and sorted into discrete categories. Our sensory perceptions of light and touch and taste, our kinesthetic feedback as we move from place to place or task to task, our memories of the people involved at every event during the day and how we would normally interact with them, all of these things are jumbled to some degree now as the boundaries we have erected in Earth-consciousness no longer exist on Altzair. As you described, in one moment your mind is clear and you are with old friends. In the next, you are with strangers and it doesn't make sense or is even threatening for them to be so close or acting so familiar with you."

Patrick has been listening uncomfortably as Alice finishes.

"I really feel like I am part of the problem here. Instead of helping, I find myself frustrated and critical of Julie when she doesn't seem to remember even the most basic things, like how to behave in church or how to be nice to one of our close friends. Part of me knows she cannot control what is happening here while at the same time I am upset with her when she is not in control."

Julie: "Yes, and I can feel your frustration. It seems like you are either frustrated or patronizing or both. How much fun is that?"

Alice: "There are two behaviors I want you to think about for a moment, *pushing* and *letting go*. Pushing represents our everyday, controlling, left-brain behaviors where trying harder and expending more effort allows us some degree of success in shaping what is happening in our life. If I work harder and faster, there is a reward waiting somewhere for me. Right? Patrick, if you do everything you can to support Julie with your time and energy and love, you expect this to have an effect that makes a real difference. Correct? Spending more time with Julie, reading about Alzheimer's, managing your conversations, being aware of the subtleties in consciousness and human interaction, adding new medications, all of this will make a difference—or will it?

"The problem with Alzheimer's is that in the left-brain realm you do have very little control. And, the idea of 'pushing' to make something happen brings with it an unintended consequence: evaluation. Because pushing carries with it the idea of focused, intentional behavior (I intend to be successful in this endeavor), it also includes an analysis of whether or not this behavior accomplished your objectives. In Julie's case, it is difficult not to evaluate how well she is functioning, compared to 'normal,' what she remembers, and how well the two of you are communicating. The catch here is that just the idea of evaluation, even if you never focus on it directly, changes the nature of your interaction. The entire sequence of behavior has a cause-effect flow to it because you were expecting something to happen."

Julie: "Do you know where I really feel you pushing Patrick?"

Patrick: "Memory?"

Julie: "Exactly! How many times a day do you ask me if I remember something?"

Patrick: "Obviously too many, I guess."

Alice: "What you are describing is very common for families in the early to middle stages of the Alzheimer's process and may be present in the later stages. It is called the 'memory test.' You Patrick are checking to see how Julie is doing and the obvious test is to check her memory of things that were familiar to both of you. Just by checking and saying something like 'do you remember ...,' you are also clearly evaluating Julie. The memory test is a classic example of

74

how to destroy quality time together by focusing on something other than the present."

Julie: "I hate it because, even though I know Patrick means well, just trying to remember is often stressful for me. Being in church or our weekly meetings with friends are even worse because I often cannot remember the names or my connection with the people present."

Alice: "Social situations such as church or a dinner with friends and any other traditional form of get-together are especially difficult because it isn't just you, Patrick, who are evaluating Julie, it is the whole set of friends or colleagues that you are with. And to make matters even worse, most social settings bring with them their own rules and expectations. So, in church, Julie not only is dealing with friends and their expectations, she is also expected to remember a fairly complex protocol that involves many different steps or stages in time—now you sit, now you sing, now you rise, now you listen. For someone with Alzheimer's, this is a worst-case scenario. Walking through a set of steps that don't make sense and wondering, when you take a step, why you are there. Not much fun.

"Letting go' is just the opposite. It is a state of mind that is coming from a more spiritual or meditative place where the world is not a thing to be pushed and controlled but rather a place where events are simply revealed, in the moment. These events or experiences don't depend on you controlling things; instead they are flowing along at their own pace. You can be part of this flow or, if you are still in controlling mode, you can resist the flow. When you share Earth-reality with someone, you are sharing a world where by consensual agreement, the events in that world come with certain rules or expectations you both understand. Sitting in church together is a good example. In this reality, pushing to be sure that your behavior or that of a friend follows the expected protocol is a type of social 'tuning' that we all learn. Being in church is like tuning to K-GOD on the radio. Everyone who tunes in gets roughly the same message. When you, Patrick, are still in Earth-reality but dealing with a friend or partner with Alzheimer's, pushing doesn't make any sense. You have to allow Julie's behavior, unless it endangers her, to follow its own path, which of course, as you already know, it will, because you cannot control it. This is the meaning of 'letting go.' Julie's world is less and less a shared, left-brain reality and more and more a world that you can only choose to accept and be part of the flow or resist and be continually frustrated.

"I don't recommend resisting. It will make both of your lives miserable; but remember—you have a choice."

Patrick: "Thank you Alice. I can see that I am putting a lot of pressure on Julie."

Alice: "The blessing that 'letting go' brings is that it adds slack to your interactions, which in turn adds many precious long moments."

Patrick: "Slack?"

Alice: "One of my favorite terms. We give each other slack when we accept whatever the other person offers without judgment. You can be too loud, like rock music when I don't, need a shower, be manic in hot weather, put too much garlic on your potatoes, or whatever, and this will not change my affection for you because I am giving you lots of room to be whatever you want to be. That is slack and unless she is endangering herself, Julie will need this gift from you.

"When you go home today, I have a simple exercise for both of you.

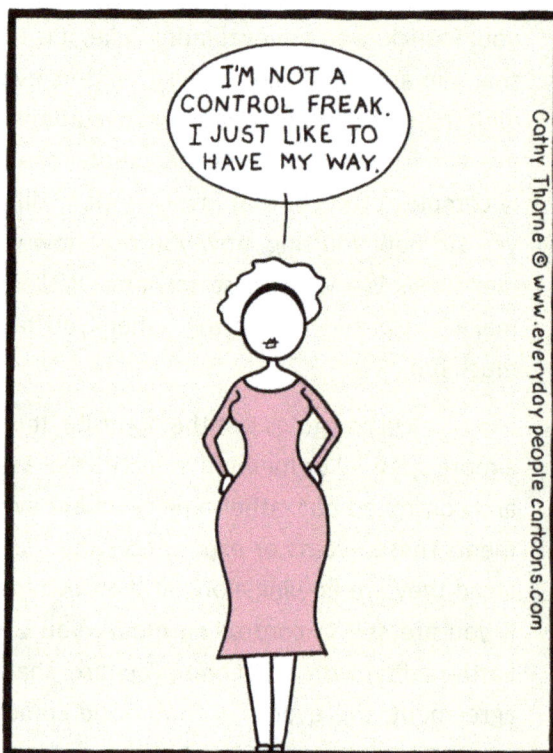

"Julie, you have permission to follow your mind, wherever it takes you, in the moment. When it takes you down familiar pathways in Earth-time that is fine. From simple tasks such as dressing or bathing or dining to complex ones such as meeting friends or completing a project, you are to enjoy these long moments while they are still available to you. On the other hand, you also have permission to visit Altzair whenever you want. You may not initiate a visit consciously, but you know the feelings that tell you that you have crossed over into that other world: the confusion, the anxiety, perhaps a sense of paranoia, all of the things that tell you something is wrong. What I want you to begin to say to yourself is that nothing is wrong, my anxiety is coming from not being in control as I leave Earth-reality, and I don't need to really change anything or fix anything. God and the universe are part of me and will help release the fear I am experiencing if I will simply let it go.

"Two things will happen as you begin to repeat these statements to yourself. First they will gradually begin to impact the quality of the time you are spending on Altzair so it is less stressed and you are under less pressure to conform to the rules of our shared Earth-reality. Secondly, as you spend more and more time on Altzair and begin to lose your ability to connect with earth reality so that these self-talk conversations become more difficult and less frequent, you will have done a wonderful thing for your unconscious mind. Your self-talk will have trained it! And now it can help communicate to you that it is OK to be on Altzair and to let go of the fear and conflicts you may otherwise be experiencing. As Alzheimer's progresses, long moments depend more and more on the unconscious mind because it will feed the dreams that will more and more become your experiences.

"If we look back historically and watch the evolution of human consciousness over time, we see that early human consciousness was probably much more direct and tied to what you were experiencing, not self-talk. If you saw a bear, you were dealing with the bear, not an abstract set of statements or words about the bear. During the course of Alzheimer's disease, the mind loses its ability to deal with these abstract verbal conversations in your head and is more like the mind of your ancestors, dealing with the experience of 'now' without words to interpret it, rationalize it, or relate it to an abstract *you* who is in some way separated from the experience.

"Finally, I want to say something to both of you. You are beginning a long journey with many unfamiliar stops along the way. Please ask for help. There will be many times you don't have the answer. You are not alone. Many others have been down a similar path and you can learn from their experiences. I am here to offer guidance as is this institution, but you will find many others waiting to assist you as well. When you need help, please be active and ask."

---

*Please see John Zeisel's excellent book, *I'm Still Here*, for further details on what memories remain in Alzheimer's patients, some keys for meaningful communication and how to connect using the arts.

HEAR MY VOICE

The Institution

I know in my heart that it will soon be time for me to leave our home and move to an institutional setting. My behavior is simply too erratic, paranoid, hostile, or unpredictable for you to manage and also have a life of your own. I forgive you for making this change to care for me despite the difficulties that it will cause. You see, for you, moving from room to room in our house, going to the office, travelling downtown on the subway, visiting a hospital or a store is OK and familiar because you immediately adapt to the different look and feeling of the environment and understand the different functions and rules associated with the environment. But I no longer have this ability.

Our home to me is much more than a place to live. It is a place that speaks to me in its own language, every day, about my intentions at any moment and how I might fulfill them. With its familiar rooms and objects and functions, it offers constant landmarks to help me navigate the day. As my speech functions and normal left-brain processing of the world disappears, this home environment has grown more and more important.

When you move me, I will be angry and upset. I will probably not understand fully why we are moving and that the move is an act of love and kindness and consideration on your part. Please forgive me for this behavior. I cannot control it. What you may not know is that without constant monitoring and support by you for some period of time the move may send me into a spiral that accelerates the symptoms of Alzheimer's disease and causes me to lose hope. Unlike you who can adapt quickly to almost any new environment, this change for me is more like a horror movie where suddenly I am imprisoned and while the guards act pleasant they have a new, sinister agenda that is not revealed to me.

Research shows that many individuals with dementia or advanced Alzheimer's don't survive a move to a hospital or an institution. I plan to survive but I will need lots of support from you to make the transition.

The Alzheimer's Cards can help here. Please use them as often as possible to help anchor me and deal with my fears. When you cannot communicate with me, they can be my voice.

Chapter 7: The Planet Altzair

The idea of you and your partner or friend with Alzheimer's living in different realities is one that your common sense and experience suggest may be correct, but conceptually, it is not obvious what this really means. You are both actually living on Earth, breathing the same air, eating the same kinds of food, and watching the same sun rise in the morning and set in the evening. Yes, Alzheimer's has impacted your partner's mental functioning to the point where they are not functioning well in the world that we share, but this world hasn't changed. A tree is still a tree, a rock is a rock. Right? The Earth and the reality it represents is still the same.

To address these questions, I have a simple exercise for you to consider.

Agreements

Early in the book I introduced the idea that we all share agreements about reality, especially social reality, and that it is these agreements that, to a large degree, define what is real, *not* a collection of immutable physical principles. Of course we do live in a world governed by physical laws such as gravity, thermodynamics, mass, and momentum, as well as all of the physics that underlies the functioning of our biological systems. However, unless our interaction with these physical systems is extreme or in some way unique, we ignore them. Gravity impacts all of us in a consistent way regardless of whether we have Alzheimer's disease, another disorder, or are perfectly healthy, but, until you fall off the chair, you will probably not notice it. Warmth is generally perceived as good while the excessive heat of a fire (as in a house on fire) is a danger sign. Physical pain is another common experience that is both shared and meaningful in a healthy mind and a mind battling Alzheimer's disease.

The sharing I am describing in this book is tied to social agreements, not our basic physical environment: how we treat one another; what behaviors are kind, loving, threatening, intelligent, friendly, unacceptable, or confusing; how we function in different social settings such as home, school, work, travel, sports, and many, many others; and how we interpret words or language in each of these settings. To understand how important and powerful these agreements are, just consider your reactions when someone doesn't agree or understand. What about the homeless person who comes too close or smells because they have not bathed for several months, or the person who begins to yell or cry uncontrollably in a public setting, or the con artist who is manipulating you by taking advantage of your tendency to respect certain agreements (such as the assumption that people are generally honest)?

Much of your experience, from the time you were an infant on through kindergarten, school, graduation, work, marriage, aging, and so forth, is based on social agreements. You are taught how to interpret what is happening and how to respond. Certain foods, for example, are acceptable or unacceptable in cultures across the world not because they are physically good or bad for you but because the culture has adopted them. In my family, we celebrate Christmas with raw oysters, a Southern tradition, but one that in many other regions of the United States is considered bizarre and even unhealthy. How you manage conflict is likely to be driven by your cultural background. In my spouse's family, they yelled and got over it. In my family you turned the other cheek and did everything possible to avoid conflict. Hurt feelings over a disagreement could last for weeks.

A social agreement is really just an understanding that we share about events in the world that makes them "real" because of the agreement. The definition of a sin is a classic example of one of the earliest and most important social agreements. But, if a social agreement is real, how real is it compared to other things such as the physical "law of gravity" or a physical object such as a tree. To understand this more clearly, do the following exercise.

Take a sheet of paper and draw a line down the left-hand side that goes from top to bottom. At the top of the chart write "Extremely Real" and on the bottom write "Less Real" or "Not So Real." Now, take five minutes to list everything you can think of that is part of your world, ranging from the tree outside to your best friend to the dream you had last night. Where do they fit on the chart?

Most likely physical items such as the tree or your car or gravity fit near the top of your chart. Dreams, ghosts, and unicorns are perhaps closer to the bottom. But you will also notice that most social agreements—about love, colors, intimacy, God, food, work, the legal system, and so forth—are also very near the top of the chart, just below the physical items.

Ultimately, looking at your chart, I would probably have to conclude that in your world many social agreements are quite "real." "Yes," you say, "no big deal. What is your point?"

The point is a simple one but a crucial one for understanding Alzheimer's disease and how it impacts personality. If much of your reality is based on shared agreements about the world, what happens when your partner can no longer share with you? What happens when, in their world, the agreement is no longer meaningful, not because they deliberately cast it aside but because the disease attacks the connections in the brain that made the agreements work. Remember from chapter 5 that a sequence of behaviors tied together logically and directed toward some goal is very challenging for someone with Alzheimer's. At their core, social agreements are largely shared, logical constructions in the mind that we use to filter the events of the world into categories so we can interpret them. As the mind loses its capacity to process logical events that extend across a period of time, it loses much of its ability to interpret and act on many of our shared agreements. In other words, it loses connection with much of what is "real" in our Earth-space. Yes, gravity still operates, but "until further notice," any shared agreements may not be valid.

> Norma has been a resident at Mom's nursing home for a number of years. I learned from the aides that she is from Kentucky but moved to Florida to be close to her daughter. Norma has Alzheimer's with a vivid imagination. She is extremely loud and vocal, sometimes sings "Row, Row, Row Your Boat" or "Jesus Loves Me." Occasionally she will begin a song like "My Old Kentucky Home," but gets the words all tangled and then gets very frustrated and just yells. One Sunday while visiting Mom, I noticed that Norma was visibly upset. I went over to where she was seated and asked her what was wrong. She turned to me in anguish and said, "Little Boy Blue is dead, he fell in a well." I simply did not know how to answer her at that point. Had nursery rhymes become real or was there a tragedy in her past? I couldn't get this off my mind. As I was leaving, I asked the nurse on duty about Norma's past, and she assured me that Norma was not relating to anything in her life, but to the nursery rhyme characters that had become real to her.

A quick look at the current state of physical science may help here. Physical reality—the rocks, the planets, the trees, the laws of motion, the sun, and, of course, the universe of atomic particles and the world we construct around them—are very real. Correct? Well, yes and no. Until the twentieth

century, the answer would have been a resounding "yes" that most scientists supported. There is a small problem with this model, however, that it took recent developments in quantum mechanics to resolve. While traditional physics works well locally (imagine a map of Kansas City that you are using to navigate where you can use a ruler to find the shortest route between two points), it does not work well on a larger scale (imagine a map of the Earth's curved surface where a straight line is no longer the shortest point). In fact, what quantum mechanics suggests is that the current world we are experiencing is only one of many possible worlds that we might be experiencing.

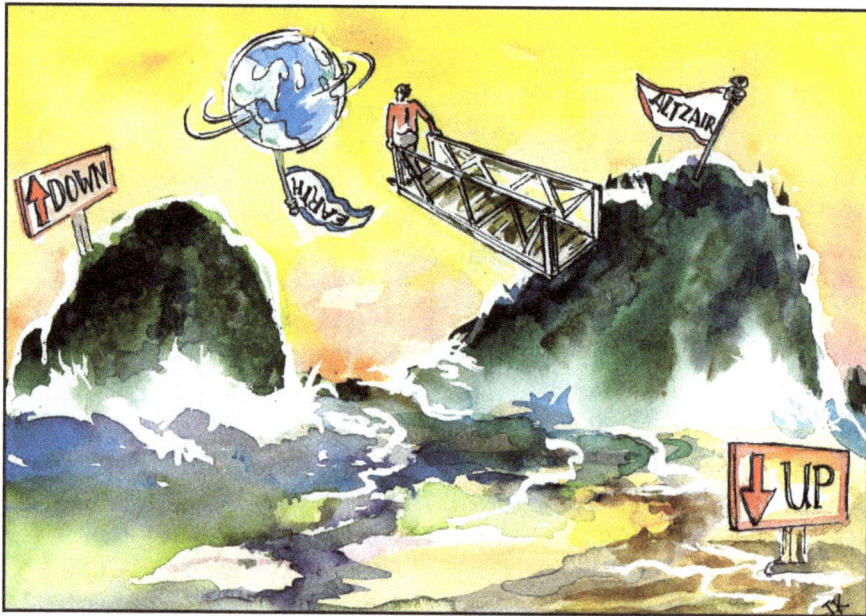

Returning to Earth from the planet Altzair can be very difficult!

This is not a bad description of the experience your friend with Alzheimer's is currently having. Some time ago their world began to diverge from yours. The rules of that world, especially those rules that tie to shared agreements in Earth-time, no longer apply. The straightedge that used to work so well to measure distances in Kansas City no longer works on Altzair. In this alien landscape, there are many precious long moments which, in a small local area, you and your friend can still share; but, at the larger or macro level, you cannot put the genie back into the bottle. The planets have already diverged. Any events outside of this unique long moment when you are both in the present and together are likely to be distorted when viewed from one world looking at the other.

Where do these worlds overlap? We know that the Alzheimer's patient is living in the present, in the moment. We know that the conversations we take for granted in Earth-consciousness where we can talk to ourselves and use words and abstract concepts as a substitute for reality are no longer possible. We know that the connections between all of our thoughts and actions and the continuous flow of time has been disrupted. We know that in some respects living in the present on Altzair simplifies consciousness (with no past or future to complicate things) but that we are still dealing with an adult mind filled with experiences and emotions, not the mind of a child. How can we describe what is happening here?

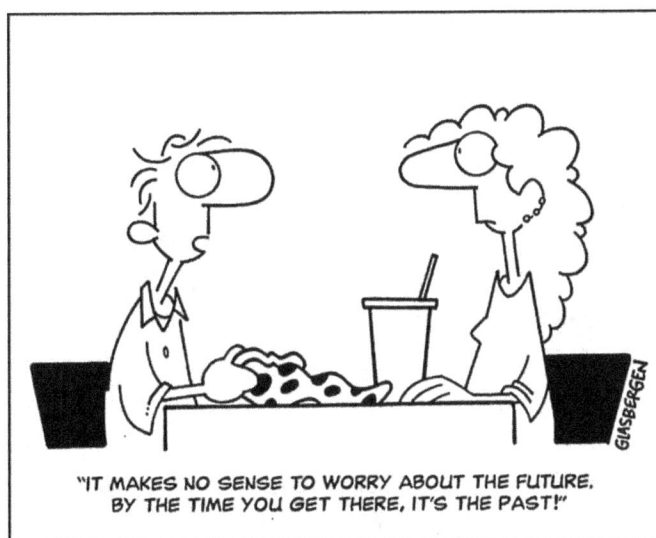

"IT MAKES NO SENSE TO WORRY ABOUT THE FUTURE.
BY THE TIME YOU GET THERE, IT'S THE PAST!"

In many respects, Alzheimer's disease represents a march back in evolutionary time to a place where the talking part of the mind no longer is in control of consciousness and where intuition, emotions, and images play a stronger role. The events of the day are no longer an abstraction (or Plato's shadows) dancing on a wall for us to view and manipulate with language. Sunset, for example, is not an idea that can be treated intellectually and planned around ("let's sit on the porch and have cocktails at sunset today"). Instead, sunset is often perceived as a somewhat unexpected, disturbing event that can produce anxiety and unpredictable reactions. It is daytime and suddenly, without warning, the light begins to wane and it grows dark outside! Biologically this is *not* a benign process. The mind of the Alzheimer's patient is living in a much more primitive biological space where ending the day can bring on fear and uncertainly. Remember in the movie *50 First Dates*, Lucy began each day fresh without memory of the previous day. In middle and late state Alzheimer's disease, this is a common experience. The individual is living so much in the moment that there is no history of experiences over time. Yesterday and much of long-term memory is damaged and inaccessible. There is no history of "sunset" as a daily event that can be anticipated. It is a new experience made even more powerful because of its strong connections to our biological clock.

Katherine was sitting with Emilou at the dining table helping her with lunch. Nearby, Stanley was sitting with Mary, his younger spouse. Mary's frustration was evident as she pummeled Stanley with questions and repeatedly received confused, unsatisfactory answers. Stanley kept glancing to his left toward Katherine, who finally stepped over, said hello to Mary, and took his hand. Relief flooded his face as he bowed his head, closed his eyes, and quietly wept.

In the early stages of Alzheimer's disease, there is still much sharing of experiences in time and a history, so long moments can contain elements that are common to shared Earth-reality. Later, however, the frequency of these shared moments on Earth will be less and less and sharing will be all about the present flavored with the past but only as it is being experienced on Altzair. And life on Altzair can be very confusing to an outsider! Think of it like a damaged film that is playing in your mind. Parts of that film will appear to touch Earth-reality and look familiar—for example, your friend with Alzheimer's is with her mother on vacation—that sounds pretty normal. Actually no, remember that this is a damaged film and just because you, the caregiver, recognize some of these situations, you cannot for a moment imagine what is really happening. This is the planet Altzair, after all. The idea of your friend's mother is certainly familiar, but what your friend is experiencing is not your version (or the Earth-reality version) of mother and vacation with mother, it is rather a whole new experience distorted by the warped perspective of all experiences on Altzair. The memory and experience on Altzair may appear to be benign and enjoyable, but still, it is a dream transformed by the bad seed of Alzheimer's disease, not a memory you can relate to in Earth-reality.

84

Long moments that involve some mix of the present with dreams from Altzair are common in middle and late stage Alzheimer's disease. When you listen to these dreams, as the caregiver, there is no reason to discourage them because they often contain anchors that connect to healthy areas of the mind.

In this context, when there is no judgment of the accuracy of the experience then music, work, hobbies, sports, and many other kinds of activities can offer richness and joy in the moment. Your friend's kinesthetic memory will retain much of the experience of riding a bike, for example. Auditory memory will recall a favorite tune, not in the sense that you can talk about it to yourself but that will connect it to feelings and experiences not in your conscious mind. These kinds of memories can be very stimulating, in a healthy way, when they are accepted without evaluation.

How do you increase the chances of this happening? Think of bubbles in a tank of water gently rising to the surface. Some of the bubbles carry messages in your shared reality. Most don't. After all, they

I watched with much interest as the new science building was constructed at TCU. It was a beautiful design with courtyards and columns and curved stairs with magnificent lighting. There was only one problem. I think it was designed to be a larger building and then downsized for cost reasons at the last minute after the physical support structure, the columns, were already in place. The result was that in the final building the columns could appear anywhere, in the middle of an office or a hallway or other unexpected places. The final design was beautiful but funky because it didn't always serve functionality. It remains one of my favorite buildings because of the many surprises!

are messages from Altzair. If your mind is free and not engaged in our typical left-brain mode of thinking where you are "pushing" to make something happen with your friend and evaluating them on whether or not it is happening (are they "having a good day" because they are communicating with me), then a marvelous thing happens. Suddenly you are fully connected with your friend's experience both on and off of Altzair. By "letting go," you become a real participant in their world, listening, aware of moments when they connect with your world, but, at the same time, aware and appreciative of them in all of the other moments when they don't connect.

The bubbles continue to rise to the surface and you allow them to reveal, without judgment, whatever messages they contain from memories of your shared experience on Earth or from Altzair. It doesn't matter. The bubbles are filled with many things, the pain and fear of Alzheimer's, a direct connection to you in this moment, confusion and uncertainty, shared memories, darkness and paranoia, love, jumbled thoughts, physical sensations of warmth and comfort, and so forth. You are relaxed, engaged, accepting of whatever comes and beginning to learn that while time still brings you shared long moments in a common reality, all long moments with your friend are in their own way precious. Your presence in these moments while your friend is on Altzair offers another kind of connection and comfort to your friend. Your willingness to open other channels of communication through touch and acceptance and gentle caring emotions brings the blessing of peace, a blanket that can temporarily sooth the raging inferno in your friend's mind that is the reality of Alzheimer's.

Listening, not judging, communicating in the channels that remain largely untouched by the disease ... these are precious gifts to your friend. But they are only part of the solution.

Shared agreements and the underlying social and physical reality that you share depend on structure. How to make a sandwich is about a structured sequence of steps that take place in a physical environment, the kitchen, in a specific order. As Alzheimer's progresses, both the sequence and the meaning of the steps in the sequence are likely to be distorted or lost. How do you deal with this?

There are two crucial steps you need to take here. First, you create environments where the structure is built in. Second, you provide the communication tools, using the Alzheimer's Cards, needed to give individuals some control over these environments using your assistance as the facilitator.

Thinking about obvious environmental manipulations to add structure, I am reminded of the airports or government buildings with big arrows on the floor to direct users to the right terminals or offices, or the best websites that grab a user and guide them, step by step, though some process (usually one that leads to a charge on your credit card). The structure of the environment for your friend or partner with Alzheimer's needs to function in a similar manner. Since the mental images of the correct sequence may be lost for many behaviors, the role of the mind here needs to be replaced by environment cues whenever possible. A drawer in the refrigerator labeled "lunch" immediately helps the person with Alzheimer's orient correctly to the right area versus opening the door and not remembering why.

To a person living on Altzair, what was once a familiar and friendly environment quickly becomes one that can be challenging to navigate because while the components may still be familiar (yes, I recognize that stove and refrigerator), the rules that connect these components to behavior can no longer be taken for granted. We can all remember the environments—a school, an airport, a hotel, a police station, an office—where we didn't have a clue about where to go or what actions to take. I am reminded of the subway systems in Paris or London where at first it was difficult for me to orient and understand which signs to follow in part because there are so many unfamiliar signs.

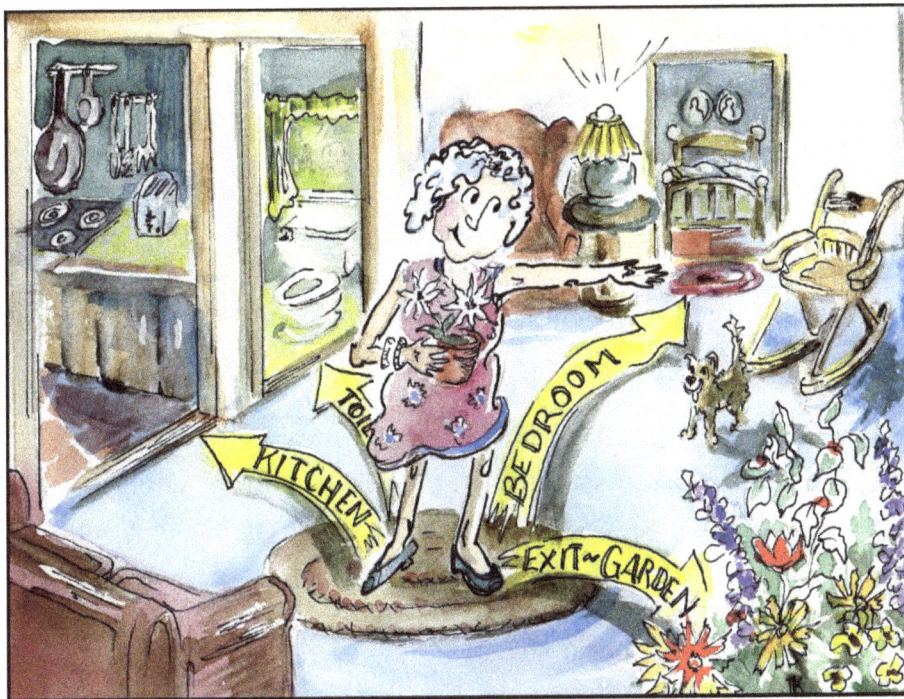

Which path shall I take? I think I will head outside to the garden.

Compare my experience in Paris to the typical user experience on a well-designed website today where each step is identified and the options are to "continue" to the next step or go back. I can still mess things up, but it is much more difficult to get off track with the helpful instructions on every screen. A well-designed environment for a person with Alzheimer's disease can benefit from this approach so that wherever he or she looks they always see cues to remind them of appropriate actions.

For many years I worked as an environmental psychologist creating designs that worked in institutional settings such as hospitals, schools, clinics, and public housing. The core idea here was to blend the traditional architectural and economic approaches to design, which are more about aesthetics and cost, with a functional approach that focuses on the needs and requirements of the users. The central issue here, as I quickly learned, watching some elegant designs (from the designer's perspective) fail miserably in real world settings, is control. If the design allows the user to function in a manner that makes them competent or successful or happy in the environment, generally that is regarded as a design that worked. If the design interferes with or impedes user functionality, then it doesn't work.

Individuals with Alzheimer's disease need control. John Zeisel identifies eight key areas where managing the environment can help:

- Exits: Need to be clearly marked and not camouflaged
- Walking Paths: Need to encourage going to a destination versus wandering
- Privacy: Personal spaces with mementos support safety, security, and familiarity
- Shared Spaces: Designs that help identify and differentiate the functions of each space guide the user
- Gardens: Need contact with nature in a safe, controlled setting
- Homelike Spaces: Create familiar, homelike settings in an institutional environment with art, furniture, and design
- Five Senses: Environments that stimulate all of our senses provide helpful clues for functioning
- Independence/Empowerment: Use designed elements to empower people by allowing them to function independently

All of these suggestions, as you can see, are actually about empowerment and control. The design guides behavior by offering clues, which are always present and speak to the purpose of the space, the walkway, the equipment, or the entrance/exit. The changes in design allow a stranger from Altzair to still function well physically on the Earth. The sense of being in control here reduces stress and in turn facilitates more opportunity for long moments that bring joy or stimulation to the present.

The second step here is to facilitate control through communication. How does a person who can sense the environment is not working or who has a need to change the environment—but cannot tell you this in a normal conversation—get this message across to you? In designing the Alzheimer's Cards, I included a section on the environment with cards such as "I am COLD," "I want to be OUTSIDE," "It's too DARK in here," and "I want to have more PRIVACY." These simple cards and others you can design yourself for a friend with Alzheimer's disease offer at least a small measure of control by simply allowing the individual to communicate their needs.

Healthy people living in Earth-reality often take the environment for granted because if it is not working for them we can quickly change it. Alzheimer's patients are largely trapped in their environments and certainly in many settings victimized by the lack of people-friendly design. A few simple changes to add structure, as described above, or tools to open communication channels can make a huge difference in the well-being of these patients.

From the private journal of J.D. Michaels, "Descending into Darkness"

The Garden: Today when Shelia visited we sat in the garden. I love the orderliness of the garden. My world now is such a kaleidoscope of events all jumbled together from morning to night that typically we can share very little of our separate worlds. But, the garden is different. I always feel as if I belong there. There is peacefulness to the rows of flowers, the trees, the paths, and the bench where we sat. It is almost like writing. How can I write these words, you are wondering, and not remember what I wrote fifteen minutes ago?

Easy, I sit at my computer, read the last page of my journal on the screen, recover some parts of the context and flow, and then, continue writing. The words just come, like now. I don't edit them or censor them, they just come. When I started keeping the journal, there was a pattern in my mind that connected the days, but this doesn't seem to be happening now. I am here, I am writing, and the words represent what is in my mind "now," not my history. The page, the computer, the words create an order that I love. It is like the garden with the rows of plants and walkways. I don't need to know why I am there. It just brings me peace.

HEAR MY VOICE

Using the Alzheimer's Cards

Practice with the Alzheimer's Cards is helpful and necessary to be sure that as Alzheimer's progresses they continue to remain relevant and keep a window open to planet Altzair for as long as possible. A "spread" of the cards simply means allowing the person to connect the cards with a specific set of things in their life. I think the HOW AM I DOING spread described below offers a good basic communication device for some individuals.

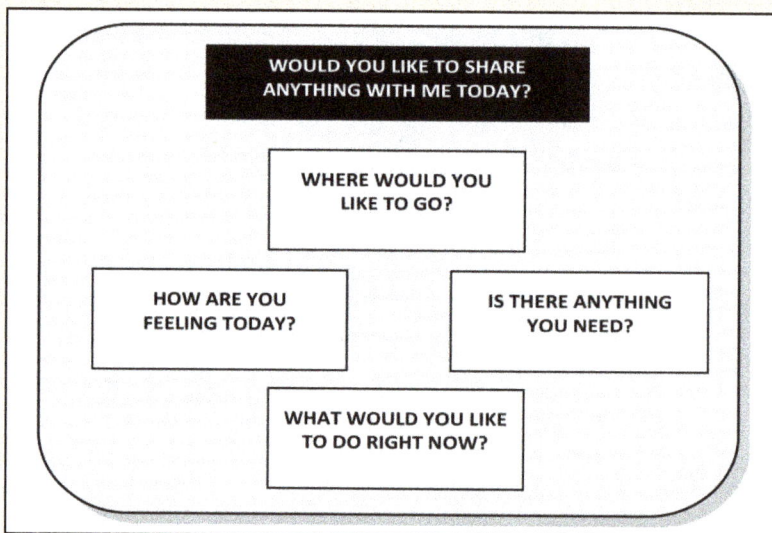

```
┌──────────────────────────────────────────────────┐
│   ╭────────────────────────────────────────╮     │
│   │   ┌────────────────────────────────┐   │     │
│   │   │  WOULD YOU LIKE TO SHARE       │   │     │
│   │   │  ANYTHING WITH ME TODAY?       │   │     │
│   │   └────────────────────────────────┘   │     │
│   │         ┌──────────────────┐           │     │
│   │         │  WHERE WOULD YOU │           │     │
│   │         │  LIKE TO GO?     │           │     │
│   │         └──────────────────┘           │     │
│   │  ┌──────────────┐   ┌──────────────┐   │     │
│   │  │ HOW ARE YOU  │   │ IS THERE     │   │     │
│   │  │ FEELING      │   │ ANYTHING     │   │     │
│   │  │ TODAY?       │   │ YOU NEED?    │   │     │
│   │  └──────────────┘   └──────────────┘   │     │
│   │      ┌──────────────────┐              │     │
│   │      │ WHAT WOULD YOU   │              │     │
│   │      │ LIKE TO DO       │              │     │
│   │      │ RIGHT NOW?       │              │     │
│   │      └──────────────────┘              │     │
│   ╰────────────────────────────────────────╯     │
└──────────────────────────────────────────────────┘
```

Always start by asking "What do you want to share with me today?" Let them select a card. Then select the next four cards using the template above. You can change the words so they fit your style here.

Your job is just to listen and acknowledge what they are telling you with their choices. If you have been using the deck for awhile, the connections between the cards will be obvious to you. In some cases a specific choice may lead you to ask questions to get more information—and occasionally take some action. Normally though you are listening and honoring what is communicated without trying to problem solve or take an action.

Note: This is an exercise for early/middle stage Alzheimer's patients using the cards designed for them. It is very likely to be too complex for late stage patients!

Chapter 8: Margie and Maxine

Maxine: *"I'm so sorry. I can feel the darkness descending on me. Why are you here today? My heart and body tell me that I know you, but my conscious mind tries and tries to connect you with my life and cannot. Are you a friend? No, now I remember. You are my life partner. Why are we meeting here instead of our home?*

"I know that you are struggling because I am here. You need my help and presence in your life for our business and our family to be successful. I know that I have let you down. I miss living with you. You have spent most of our savings to care for me in this nice facility. I'm so sorry. I have let you down. I don't understand. There don't seem to be any options. The curtains are closing in my mind, in my world. How do I get out of the way? I'm angry and afraid at the same time.

"I am dreaming much of the time now as my mind struggles to distinguish between what is real and what is imaginary. You and I went on a picnic yesterday. We were at our summer cabin in the Adirondacks. It was wonderful to be with you again. Part of me knew that this could not be possible, that we are both much older, but the dream has become my reality now and so your presence was very real for me. Grandmother joined us on the lake, then our friends Dick and Martha from here in Cincinnati, then the lake was filled with beautiful yachts from Nice and the smell of chocolate and oranges, and then it was night and I was alone and afraid."

Alice: "It is good to see you today Margie. Have you visited with Maxine yet?"

Margie: "No, not yet, I was hoping to chat with you for a moment before I went to her room."

"Of course," replies Alice. "What is on your mind?"

"I feel like she is slipping away from me very rapidly now. She can often still recognize me, but not remember who I am, and if she does remember, it is connected with some imaginary situation she has created in her mind. It's bizarre and makes me feel very uncomfortable. I don't know how to respond."

"I'm sorry. I know how difficult it is to lose a companion that you have known and loved most of your life. Perhaps I can help you understand what she is experiencing and, in turn, this can help you come from a more comfortable place when you are with her.

"Imagine that Alzheimer's is like a seed that was planted in Maxine's mind, many years ago. The seed represents a model of reality, but it is a model not grounded in Earth-reality in any way. Think of it as a rather bad Earth-model where memories and rules for how to get along in the world and experiences are all jumbled together in a somewhat haphazard manner. We have talked about this before as being on the planet Altzair."

"Yes, I remember."

"As the seed grows, it becomes a larger and larger part of Maxine's mind and begins to dominate her consciousness. Because the seed really is just a bad model of her mind, it has the same people, the same memories, the same experiences as exist in her healthy mind. The problem is not just that all of this is jumbled together in a chaotic manner, but much worse: Maxine cannot separate the parts of reality she is experiencing that are just memories created by the seed from what is actually valid in the Earth-reality she is sharing with you.

"What this means is that every moment of her life is filled with a kind of insane dilemma. Her mind is filled with information, about you, her room, the TV, and all of the other things happening in her consciousness, but, unfortunately, she cannot separate the parts that are real from the parts that are dreams. She is in a dream of a dream of a dream where she is never quite sure in which one of the dreams she is actually awake. The anchors that tie these dreams

> *I remember flying back to Dallas with a retarded young man in his twenties sitting in the row opposite me excitedly talking about everything he was experiencing on the flight. When the plane landed, he erupted in a spasm of joy and delight that promptly attracted the attention of the flight attendants who yelled at him, in their formal "command" voices, to be quiet. Their anger and posture upset him and he stood up, confused by what was happening; his protests became even louder as a male attendant attempted to force him down into his seat. When the plane reached the gate, the police rushed on to escort him off.*
>
> *In that moment and many times since, I have regretted not having the courage to stand up, exchange seats with his neighbor, and put my arm around him to briefly share his joy and then, gently calm him. His experience on the plane was not unlike the experience one with Alzheimer's disease could have.*
>
> *Living with Alzheimer's disease, you are committed in ways that others, on the outside, often fear, cannot understand, and cannot control. Yet the hope is always there for your partner's touch and their commitment to be with you 100 percent with love and no evaluation.*

92

to Earth-reality are largely gone. This is part of the special hell that makes Alzheimer's such an insidious, unrelenting disease."

Margie: "How terrible. I can see some of this happening, but to listen to you describe what she is experiencing just breaks my heart. It sounds so hopeless."

"Hopeless? Yes if you are still comparing her world to your world in Earth-space. Definitely no if you begin to understand and accept the dimensions of her reality."

"How do you mean?"

"Marshal McLuhan wrote a famous book in 1964 that I think has some relevance here. Let me start with that and then I'll give you concrete examples that will help. McLuhan's book was called *Understanding Media*. The point he was making is that much of the information we receive about the world comes not from the specifics of the message—the grass is green—but rather from the channel in which we receive the message. Hearing the words, 'the grass is green,' is quite different from seeing a picture of green grass, which, in turn, is quite different from the experience of sitting in a field of green grass. McLuhan's argument is that the real message here has more to do with the channel than with the content.

> *Miss Ruth is a diminutive lady in a wheelchair who rambles non-stop all day long. If she is awake she is talking. Ruth is from South Carolina and has that endearing accent. She often sits at the same dining table as Mom, and one day when Mom and I joined Ruth at the table, she looked at Mom and asked her what grade she was in. Even in Mom's demented state, she looked puzzled and turned to me with that look that said "what?" So I smiled at Miss Ruth and asked her what grade she was in ... she promptly said seventh grade. Again, Mom looked at me with one eyebrow raised in question.*
>
> *During this brief exchange, I realized how difficult it must be for these Alzheimer patients .... Sometimes they are a child, sometimes a young housewife, a young soldier, a businessman, but others around them are in their own time zone. On this particular day, Ruth was in the seventh grade, but obviously Mom was in a different generation.*

"As you will see in a moment, the real messages you send to Maxine every time you visit absolutely have this same property. They are much more about the channel you choose than the verbal content we are so familiar with in Earth-space.

"The other point that McLuhan, Huxley, Orwell, Mander, and many others have made is that our use of media, step by step, take us from experiences in the real world to more and more abstract experiences in our mind. We move from ex-

93

periences of green grass to pictures of grass to stories about grass to conversations about grass so quickly and seamlessly and unconsciously that we often treat them as if they were all the same. Yes, I remember a field of green grass and can describe it to you in some detail, and, in the abstract world of words and ideas, you can comprehend my field of grass as part of our shared reality because, in fact, you have experienced many fields of green grass. Most of the time, however, on your visits, you are describing and remembering experiences with Maxine, unintentionally making them abstractions, rather than sharing an actual experience with her."

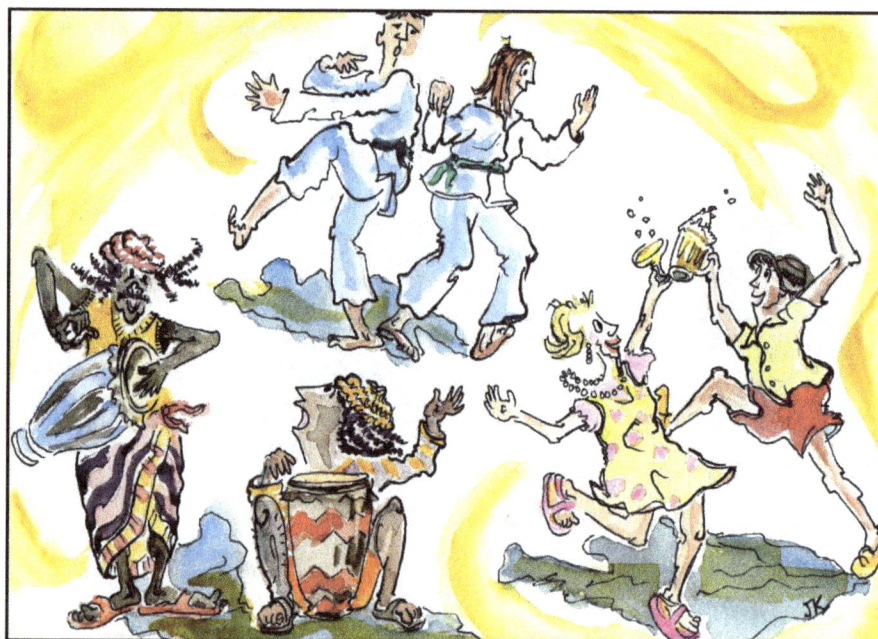

In late stage Alzheimer's while many experiences will still be remembered, the verbal descriptions of these experiences may be too abstract to be meaningful.

"I guess you are right. It is true that much of our time together has been spent talking and remembering things we shared, and while it is obvious that these memories are not the same as the experiences, we are not thinking about the difference."

"That is true for most people. Our reality for the most part is a world of words, books, TV, or the Internet, not actual experiences. The majority of people take it for granted that this is reality. Did the earthquake actually hit Japan and create a giant tsunami? Did tornados actually destroy much of Birmingham last spring? Did your friend Jill actually fall in love with the pizza delivery man? All of these things become real because we experience so much of reality in our minds.

94

My favorite way to describe this is to say that in every moment we are actually creating what we mean by reality in our consciousness.

"Earth-reality, when understood in this manner, becomes problematic for anyone suffering with Alzheimer's because the shared agreements about this reality that allow us to validate it together (think of this as tuning our versions of reality to the same channels so that we agree on how to interpret different events) become tied to more and more abstract concepts largely in our minds and not anchored to specific experiences that we have had in the world. What is an abortion like? What does it feel like to win a $1,000,000? What is it like to go into space? Most of us haven't had these experiences, but we can go to these places in our mind through a friend or the media that describes them in great detail.

"Now you can begin to see how Alzheimer's is affecting your communication with Maxine. Her mind has lost the familiar anchors in Earth-based experiences that made your shared, consensual reality possible and natural in your conversations with her. Without these anchors, memories, everyday behaviors, habits, friends, and most other things, her life is no longer solid ground for connecting her thoughts to experiences. The seed in her mind that has jumbled together experience and memory is especially by communications that are essentially about ideas or abstractions. The words that we take for granted as a representation of experience are *not* experience, just an abstract model we learned to use to describe experience. In Maxine's mind, words, experiences, and memories are mixed in a jumble of thoughts, similar to a dream, that can no longer be shared with you because many of the agreements you once had about reality are now gone."

"What is the good news here that you mentioned?"

"The good news is really very good news. Once you understand that Alzheimer's disease viscously attacks this abstract reality that is so tied to left-brain, logical thinking and self-talk, but, at the same time, leaves many other, more concrete parts of our experiences and memories intact, you are prepared to open some of these other channels. Remember the Alzheimer's seed that I mentioned a few minutes ago?"

"Of course."

"Imagine the following scenario. Once that seed is planted in the mind, it starts the dreaming process and Maxine's world or the world of anyone with Alzheimer's begins to diverge from our shared model of reality. The seed attacks the logical, rational, time-based parts of our mind most strongly, so quickly we notice these functions are compromised. As we see this happening, I would encourage you to separate the person you know, Maxine, and that person's voice from the voice of the Alzheimer's seed, the voice of the planet Altzair."

"That sounds a bit like the exorcist!"

> Miss Lucy was a precious resident who walked the halls in her very proper dresses and slippers. One day I saw her approach the nurse's station where someone had delivered a small basket of fruit. Miss Lucy announced to no one in particular that "there was her purse," she had been looking for it all afternoon. With that she promptly removed all the fruit from the wicker basket, put the handle of the basket over her arm, and strutted away down the hall.

"Yes, and truthfully, that is not such a bad analogy. Living with Alzheimer's is much like living with a devil inside of you, a voice that speaks through you but does not represent 'you,' the real person that we know and love. The voice of Altzair is truly the voice of a devil of sorts. What is fortunate though is that we can quickly learn to recognize that voice and deal with it as you already do with Maxine. And more important, you can appreciate that the real person, the Maxine you have known and loved for so many years, is still there begging for the chance to have more long moments with you.

"Let me give you another example. Suppose that in our culture we all grew up wearing red-tinted sunglasses. Image a thick red tint so that everything is colored with a red hue. You can take off the glasses, if you choose, and see other colors, but no one does this. Now imagine a special disease, 'Leaping Red Blindness.' When this disease strikes, it destroys your ability to see the color red. This is unfortunate because wearing the thick red glasses means you effectively are blind. It is very difficult and sad to lose your sight in this way, and as family and friends visit, wearing their glasses, it is frustrating for them and for you not to be able to see. One day, by accident, someone knocks off your glasses and suddenly you are seeing the world again in many other color dimensions. You are excited to tell your friends what you have discovered, but on their next visit as you try to explain, they look at you strangely and merely offer to replace the broken glasses, never accepting the fact that you could share many other versions of reality by simply using different color lenses.

96

"Maxine's mind is gradually going blind in the color red, the shared logic-based reality where we spend most of our time on the Earth. You cannot prevent this. What you can do, however, is take off the glasses and open your mind to sharing her world in the many other colors that are available."

"I don't understand, what are these other colors?"

"Let me list a few of these from Jytte Lokvig's wonderful book *Alzheimer's A to Z*. They include feelings, emotions, memories of how to do things like ride a bike or ski, life events, interactions with nature, artistic memories of music or painting, archetypical memories of major events or beliefs, religious experiences and much, much more. At every stage of Alzheimer's disease, for example, Maxine will always appreciate your smile, an emotion you can share, and things that are grounded in nature like the sun or the pool outside with goldfish.

"I have watched you learn over the past year, as you have cared for Maxine, how to not judge the logical content of what she says or try to force the conversations in a direction that makes you comfortable. Described in another way, you have learned to 'flow' with her, to be with her in the present wherever she is in her mind."

"Yes, that has been difficult to do. I keep watching for the moments when she comes back to Earth and remembers me and our life together, but, at the same time, I am much more relaxed and willing to accept wherever she is."

"Excellent, now it is time to take this idea of flow and open up the other channels of communication with her by taking off the red glasses. Maxine is still there, waiting for you in many dimensions of her mind. Waiting for your hug or smile. Waiting for your song or music or dance or laugh. Yes, the Altzair seed is still pulling at Maxine's mind, distorting reality, destroying her anchors in consensual, shared reality, but it has little effect on most other 'colors.'

"Your job is to be there with her in the present, no matter what she is experiencing. What is in her mind at any one moment is a mix of the present tense and what she is experiencing on Altzair. As you listen to her and join her flow, join her in these other dimensions but also be with her in the present. Watch for chances to take a simple statement about her brother, something she loves, something in nature she is experiencing, or any other memories and experiences not strongly impacted by Alzheimer's and turn these into long moments where you both are on the same wavelength, sharing the same colors."

"That is a lot easier said than done, Alice. Much of the time I spend with Maxine is not exactly in the 'flow.' In fact I would describe it as an uneasy silence where I am constantly looking for ways to communicate with her. Often we just sit together for an hour and don't really share anything significant."

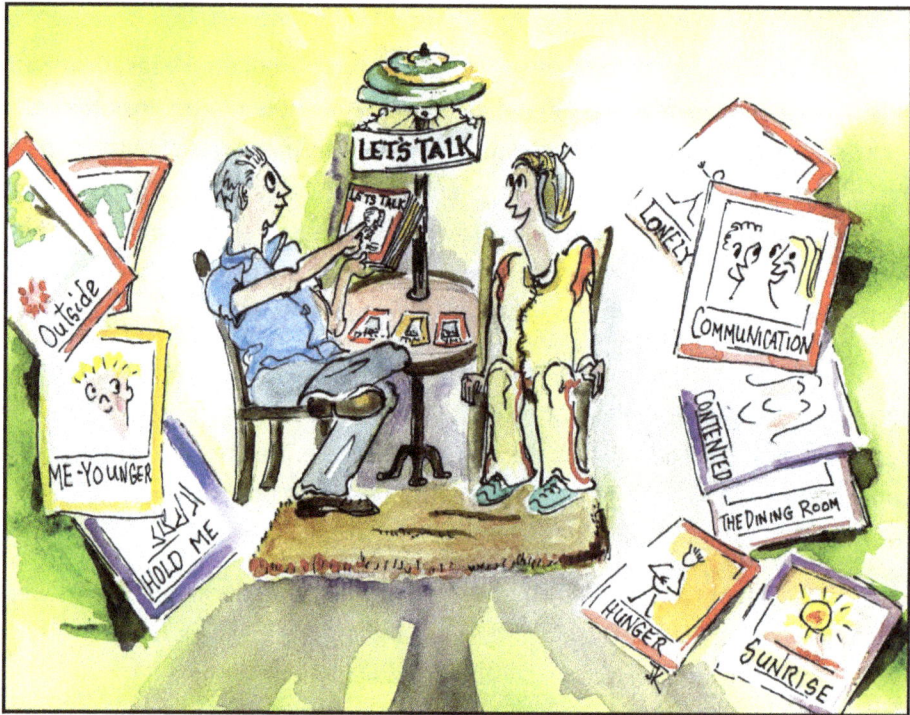

The Alzheimer's Cards offer a valuable new tool to help middle and late stage individuals communicate their needs.

"Are you using your Alzheimer's Cards with her?"

"Well, I am a little embarrassed to admit it, but no, we haven't used them for awhile. They were great aids for several years, but recently it seems that Maxine doesn't connect to the cards as strongly as she did earlier. She will recognize the pictures but the text is often too complicated for her. It seems as if the boundaries of her world have shrunk and are connected more and more with her basic needs. The ideas on the cards that made sense at one time like COMPASSION or HARMONY don't seem to connect in a meaningful way now."

"You are still using the original deck?"

"Yes, Maxine and I created it several years ago."

"It is probably time for you to shift to the deck for late stage individuals. It is a much simpler deck with just words and very simple expressions tied to needs and other basic communication. It also comes without images if you want this option. Images can be helpful at times but also, for some individuals, add confusion and complexity in the later stages of Alzheimer's disease.

"What you will find is that the process for using the late stage Alzheimer's Cards described in the accompanying booklet offers a structured protocol for administering them that helps start the communication process and enhances the chance that you and Maxine can open other channels or colors to share."

"What other channels do you recommend here?"

"The ones that work best, of course! Treat this as an experimental problem. Test the different channels and see which ones produce the best response. I recommend starting with the arts—music, painting, sculpture, dance—any of these that interest her. There are some excellent tools designed for caregivers that promote art-related exercises."

"Why the arts?"

"What you are looking for is the opportunity to bring her into the present, to create meaningful long moments with her that you can both share, even when you are on different planets. I've found over the years that the experience of the arts, especially songs or music, is something that many individuals in late stage Alzheimer's can still appreciate and respond to. The arts transcend the boundaries of our traditional, talk-oriented, evaluation-oriented left-brain consciousness similar to the way that our emotions, our spiritual life, and our experiential memory transcend these boundaries."

"That makes a lot of sense to me but will it really make any difference?"

"What do you mean?"

"Even if I do open up these other dimensions, does is really matter? Each visit it seems that Maxine has deteriorated further and my presence has less and less impact. Part of me is saying to myself "She is no longer the Maxine I know. She is a stranger. What is the point of visiting a stranger and sitting uncomfortably with them for a couple of hours?"

"You are certainly correct. Alzheimer's is an insidious, unrelenting disease process, and visit after visit Maxine will continue to deteriorate. You cannot change that."

"My point exactly."

"Now, let's take a look at where your comments are coming from. I'm going to read a few of your words back to you. How about, 'it seems that Maxine has deteriorated further and my presence has no impact.'

"Have I got that correct?"

Margie fidgets uncomfortably.

"Yes."

"What you are really saying here is about *you*, not Maxine. You are admitting that you have failed. You are not able to have the success in communicating with Margie that you hoped, and, in a typical left-brain manner, you have *evaluated* your performance and rated it as a failure. That is what is hopeless, not Margie. Am I correct?"

"Well ... I don't know. You might be right."

"If you think about this for a moment, you will know it's true. I am not evaluating you. Your family is not evaluating you. Maxine is not evaluating you. The situation is 'hopeless' only if your goal is to put the genie back into the bottle. It is frustrating and difficult for Maxine but not hopeless. Remember our earlier conversations. All of Maxine has not been impacted by Alzheimer's. Most of Maxine outside of the parts that tie to our everyday, left-brain, Earth-reality is still present. You love Maxine, as you have said many times, and want both the quality of her life and the moments she spends with you to be the best possible. Right?"

"That's correct?"

"Then it is time to move past your frustration with your own performance here caused by not sharing the same Earth-reality with Maxine and accept that she is spending most of her time now on Altzair, a completely different world. Because of this, as you have observed, she has become a stranger."

"Yes, unfortunately."

"What do you do in your everyday life when you meet a stranger? Do you ignore them and walk away because they are not familiar to you? Of course not.

What you do is you get to know them. You reach out, accept them, learn about them, and learn how to interact with them. That is where things stand now with Maxine. She is a stranger. But, she is counting on you to break down the barriers that keep her from becoming a friend and part of your life."

"That seems so artificial to me, to pretend she is a stranger. She's not a stranger. She is a friend with a disease."

"No, she is a friend certainly but a friend with a mind that has rebooted. The Alzheimer's seed has irrevocably changed her waking conscious mind and personality into that of a stranger. It's a fact and until you accept that fact and accept

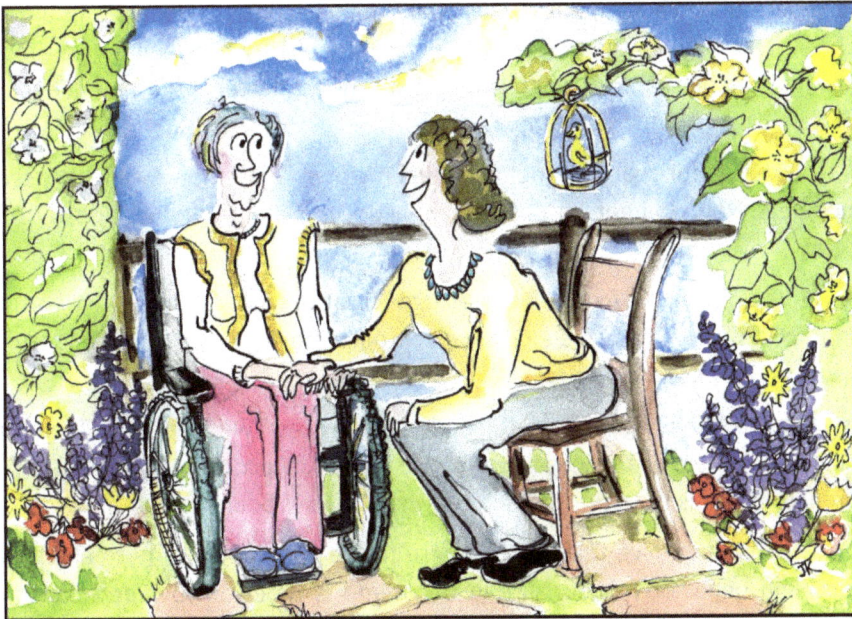

Alzheimer's means that you have me as a new friend every day, Mom.

that because she frequently sees you as a true stranger, someone she doesn't know or remember consciously, you cannot have a traditional relationship with her.

"When you walk in for a visit, you are the same old you, operating with your left brain, your self-talk, your judgmental, logical mind that wants to evaluate everything you encounter. And even when you temporarily suspend this evaluation process and attempt to flow with Maxine, you haven't become a new person. You are just a kinder, gentler, more open version of the same Margie, living in Earth-reality, who will return home after your visit and live your normal existence, in other words, you are still a stranger.

"Imagine her reaction when she doesn't recognize you—you are a true stranger—and you walk in and begin to treat her in a familiar way with a hug, holding hands, or a personal conversation."

"I know from experience, it doesn't work. She retreats from me. It can ruin my visit."

"Today when you go into the room take nothing for granted. Be sure and introduce yourself. Remind her that you are a friend who has known her for many years and that you have come to visit. If she reacts to you in a negative way, let her know that is OK and that when she is ready to talk or go outside or do anything that you might normally do on a visit, you are ready. If enough time passes you may have to introduce yourself again. Over time she will come to understand that you are her friend, now, in the present tense, and any history between you is simply a bonus that can be shared in the moment but is not expected. Your new friend lives on Altzair. Be gentle and patient."

"Thanks for coaching me. I can feel my own frustration. At times it seems so hopeless. How do I get off of this train? Poor Maxine. How does she get off of this train?"

"It's not about fixing things Margie. That is what is frustrating you. You cannot fix it. But you can take a positive approach moving beyond fear and frustration into acceptance and hope."

1. From the beginning to the end of the process, we accept our friends and family with Alzheimer's disease, we forgive them for inconveniencing us, and we remember them as the whole person they have always been and will always be.

2. We recognize that our response to the breakdown of normal left-brain speech and behavior functionality in our friend is based on *our dependency on these functions* and fear of losing them and is not a judgment of our friend. We accept and understand that once we move beyond our own fear and uncertainty here that we have no need to judge or evaluate our friend's behavior.

3. Your presence in this current situation, as a friend, spouse, or caregiver, is one of a strong, loving ally not influenced by the turbulence of the moment or society's representation of Alzheimer's as a descent into hell. Your willingness to connect with your friend on many levels of consciousness, to take communication beyond conventional left-brain chatter using experiences and the Alzheimer's Cards, and to joyfully embrace and accept this stranger who is a friend from another planet changes the rules.

HEAR MY VOICE

The Stranger

You are a stranger to me today.
Your familiarity is uncomfortable, your touch unwelcome.
I know you but that knowing is buried deep in a place
that your caring intentions can never reach.

You are a stranger to me today.
Why are you here? What do you want?
Why are you invading my space?
Please leave. Please stay. I need you so much.

You are a stranger to me today.
I have nothing to say to you. I have so much to say.
I am so frustrated. I am so helpless.
Why are you here? Please stay.

You are a stranger to me today.
Why are you here? Come closer, I want to meet you.
I know I look terrible. I am so ashamed.
Come closer, don't I know you from somewhere?

You are a stranger to me today.
But, it's OK. I'm so lonely. Will you be my friend?
Will you keep me company for awhile?
Don't I know you from somewhere?

You are a stranger to me today.
And, my friend. Welcome. Please help me.
I hurt inside and out.
I'm trapped in hell and long to be free.

You are my friend today.
My heart reaches out to you but you cannot tell.
Reach into our past and stroke me with our shared love.
And then, set me free.

—Anonymous

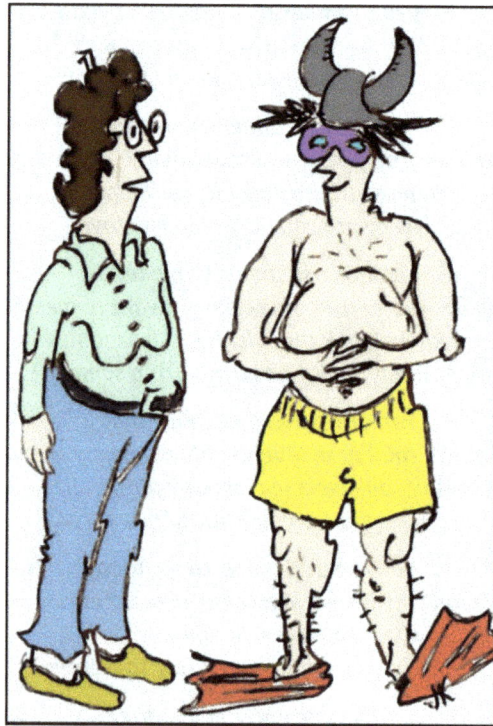

Honey, I feel like I just don't know you anymore.

Chapter 9: Late Stage Alzheimer's

In the late stages of Alzheimer's, the pull of the dream is very strong, so strong in fact that waking up may not be possible. The pull of Altzair's gravity is irresistible and the return to our normal, shared waking consciousness is no longer feasible. The seed has grown and the voice of Alzheimer's on the planet Altzair dominates all other voices, at least in the verbal, left-brain domain. Many of the simple physical anchors to Earth-reality that were connected to our everyday habits such as dining, using the toilet, dressing, or expressing basic needs have been compromised. The person may remember the habit but the logical sequence of behaviors required for even simple tasks has vanished or is distorted by the model of the world presented by the Alzheimer's seed.

If we think of time as divided into long moments, where consciousness becomes more and more focused on just the present tense and the past and future have vanished, you have a very rough idea of what the Alzheimer's patient is experiencing, with one additional twist. As the disease progresses, these moments become shorter and shorter. These are especially difficult times for friends or family members who visit only occasionally. It is a big step to go from the everyday buzz of our shared, busy, interactive reality to a world where the rules have changed so dramatically. Listening, trusting the flow of whatever is happening in the moment, and reaching out through nonverbal channels is very important, but it is just as important to understand how to experience life with someone whose world lacks the continuity in time that we take for granted in our world.

> On my visits to Mom, I have noticed a very large lady in a wheelchair holding a baby doll. She never spoke, never really seemed connected, no expressions ever. But always clung to this baby doll. When I asked about Edna, the aides said she would become very agitated and restless until they placed this doll in her arms. As soon as her arms went around the blanket holding the doll, Edna would calm down, soothe the "baby," and become comforted. How interesting to observe that Edna's Alzheimer's had her remaining in her early parenting years. While others, like Mom, drift from childhood to present day, with no lines of separation.

Have you had the experience of reaching out to shake someone's hand only to have them not respond, leaving you with your hand dangling? I remember how profound and disconcerting this simple experience can be in any context, accidental or deliberate. Visiting a late stage Alzheimer's patient can be disorienting in a similar manner. The cause-effect logic of our everyday world is gone. It is no longer a valid, operating model in this situation. I do X, you do Y, and everyone understands. This is no longer a relevant approach. Now the voices of the caregiver and patient are more like this:

The Caregiver:

"I am here for you listening and waiting. There is no hurry. I am reaching out to you in all of the emotional or physical or experiential channels that are available to us, but at the same time, I have no urgency to take you anywhere, to have you be or say anything or expect you to come back to my reality. I am waiting and watching for the opportunity to join your flow, your dream, your experience whenever you are ready."

The Alzheimer's Patient:

"You are in my space. I am annoyed and pleased at the same time. Stimulate me. Give me concrete choices. I have something to say but cannot. For me now, every moment is spent in a dark tunnel looking out at the world, which can change in a blink of the moment. Grab me in those moments and engage me."

What the missing hand example illustrates is the power of social expectations on our behavior and how quickly we become uncomfortable when these conventions are violated. Individuals in the mainstream of society are typically tied to many of these conventions. As you move toward the fringe, they become less and less relevant. If you are homeless and hungry and haven't bathed for a month, radiating an odor that is suffocating from ten feet, you may recognize that people are reacting to you in an unpleasant way but you probably also don't care. The discomfort is in the eyes of the person looking at and evaluating the homeless individual because culturally, it is probably not obvious how to respond. The same is true with Alzheimer's. It takes some practice to flow with an individual suffering middle or late stage Alzheimer's because there is a great deal of uncertainty for most people about how to behave or react. You speak to your friend and they don't respond in any predictable or conventional manner. Even though you may be expecting this, it can feel similar to the absent hand example, not comfortable.

To illustrate how different these worlds can be, consider the following example. You are visiting with your friend who has late stage Alzheimer's disease. They still recognize you as you stand in front of them. Now you slowly walk around behind them, pause a few seconds, and then return to face them again. What has happened here? In Earth-reality nothing much. You have walked around the chair and come back to where you started. On Altzair, especially in the later stages, this simple action can have profound consequences. Quite literally, you have vanished at one moment in time and then reappeared in another moment. *Welcome back to my world. What are you doing here?* Does this remind you of a magic show? It should. They are currently living in a magical world filled with uncertainty.

On Earth our twenty-four-hour cycle of night and day anchors our behaviors in time in familiar ways. Each sunrise begins a new cycle of daily routines that feed into the morning, afternoon, and then evening in a comfortable, regular manner. On Altzair, however, the planet is spinning so rapidly and erratically that the daily cycle is now reduced to moments! You can walk around your friend, disappear, and then return in a few seconds because their experience of the present may not last more than a few seconds, especially when a discontinuity occurs, like you disappearing. Imagine for a moment what a crazy, unpredictable reality your friend is forced to deal with.

Now, let's come back to the reason why you are here. What is the point of your visit? I touched on this in the last chapter because there is a tendency in all of us to make the visit about us by evaluating our performance. Remember the Alzheimer's memory test where we ask our poor friend questions to test their memory? Another version of this test in the middle or late stages is whether they remember you or remember anything about a common past like a picture, an experience, or a shared emotion. While on the surface these tests appear to be about the person with Alzheimer's disease they are just as much about you. A "good visit" means you behaved competently by interacting with your friend in such a way as to elicit past shared memories, recognition, or any form of conversation. A "poor visit" may mean you sat opposite your friend for an hour with them in a nonresponsive mode. If this happens, surely part of the problem is you not knowing what to do. Correct?

Why are you visiting in the first place? Is it like a job interview where your skills are used to extract information and conversation from the interviewee? Is the point about you feeling good about yourself because you visited and expressed your concerns by offering love or companionship for your friend? A typical hospital visit would involve the above circumstances. But not with Alzheimer's.

Your concerns and expressions of care may not even be acknowledged by the other person! Certainly this is likely to be true if you are operating in normal, everyday, Earth-based, shared-reality mode, waiting for your friend to step back into your reality.

Our everyday habits are extremely convenient because they allow us to do many routine things during the day, on automatic, without thinking. The problem is that, for an adult, they occupy 90 percent of our waking time. In an earlier book on consciousness, I encouraged readers to break the bonds that give our habits enormous control over our lives by doing a simple exercise (a discipline) to see the habit clearly, not judge or fix it. Smokers, for example, could smoke all they wanted with the catch being that when they smoked a cigarette they had to just smoke and not do anything else: no smoking with a cup of coffee or food, no smoking while driving, no smoking while watching TV. It is actually very difficult to do because our habits are not isolated but connect to many linked behaviors.

Imagine living without the comfort of habits where there is no guide or path to make the process of dressing, dining, greeting people, watching TV, reading, or doing anything else automatic. That is part of the chaos in the late stage Alzheimer's mind where there are no working programs downloaded to guide our behavior. On Altzair everything is new and needs to be processed in the moment, repeatedly, over and over.

On the other hand, if the purpose of the visit is to demonstrate caring and love for your friend, you now know that is possible through many kinds of communication channels, including use of the Alzheimer's Cards. You can come to them not expecting or waiting for them to come to you. You can be there with them sharing experiences and memories. You can help them reach into their mind and experience a long moment that is meaningful and anchored in some solid ways to their reality even if this reality is a dream in your world. A smile, a dance, music, holding hands, driving a car, being on the beach, and a thousand other memories are available that can open a window even for someone who is constantly dreaming because their mind is open to changing quickly and spontaneously with a push from an external stimulus. And finally, using the Alzheimer's Cards and listening, you can give a real voice to their feelings and needs in the moment, stimulate them with activity, and turn an hour of silence into many shared moments. What an incredible gift for your friend.

* * *

The Alzheimer's Patient:

My heart rejoices in your presence. I don't remember you in the conventional ways of remembering. I don't know your name or your history or your role in my life or even why you are here. But, I know you. My heart knows you. My body knows you. My mind knows you because you are in many of my dreams. Your presence brings forth a colophony of memories, most out of reach until you join me in remembering and celebrating them. Your touch is familiar and often comforting even if at times I react as if it is the touch of a stranger.

Your presence is very real for me even though I can no longer separate real from my dreams on Altzair. All things are real and unreal. Remember the "after death" stories we listened to with fascination? The dark tunnel and the lights leading to somewhere? My dreams are filled with darkness now. Just sitting with you in the room or outside is much like sitting in a tunnel, waiting. It feels like my world is attached to a dimmer switch and that day by day someone is rotating the dimmer a small increment toward darkness.

Joe loves to dance. As a mobile resident with Alzheimer's, Joe lives in the locked ward as he tends to wander. Oh, but every time there is music in the hall, Joe comes out dancing. He dances with the aides, the nurses, and any available visitor. One day in the dining room I was sitting with his wife as we watched several folks dancing and clapping their hands to the beat of the music. Joe was right there in the middle of it all. I turned to his wife and said, I was sure they had spent many years dancing ... But she just smiled and said, "No, we never danced. Joe has never danced, ever ... until now."

The music you play every visit now, the theme from West Side Story, *fills me with excitement. When you play that music, hold my hand, and talk quietly to me about our experiences together, the dreams are oh so sweet that I want them to continue forever. I don't mind the dark. Part of my being is in pain and struggling, as always now, part in rapture with the joy of the long moments in your presence.*

You don't owe me anything now. Our lives are on divergent paths, I know. I want you to break the bonds that hold us together and fly away. No, I want to be in your presence, always. Yes, it doesn't matter what I want. I'm on Altzair, you are on Earth. Please fly away. I love you.

* * *

Your quiet presence in love or friendship brings the most precious of gifts to your friend. Your willingness to open all channels of communication and to listen to the feedback they are giving you about touch, music, life experiences, emotions, pain, body sensations, and to respond accordingly, is a welcome gift. This is definitely not about you being an expert here or even necessarily comfortable. It is about you willing to be present, to be open, and to join your friend whenever the opportunity permits, or not; either alternative is OK. It is all about being in flow, as I described in chapter 5.

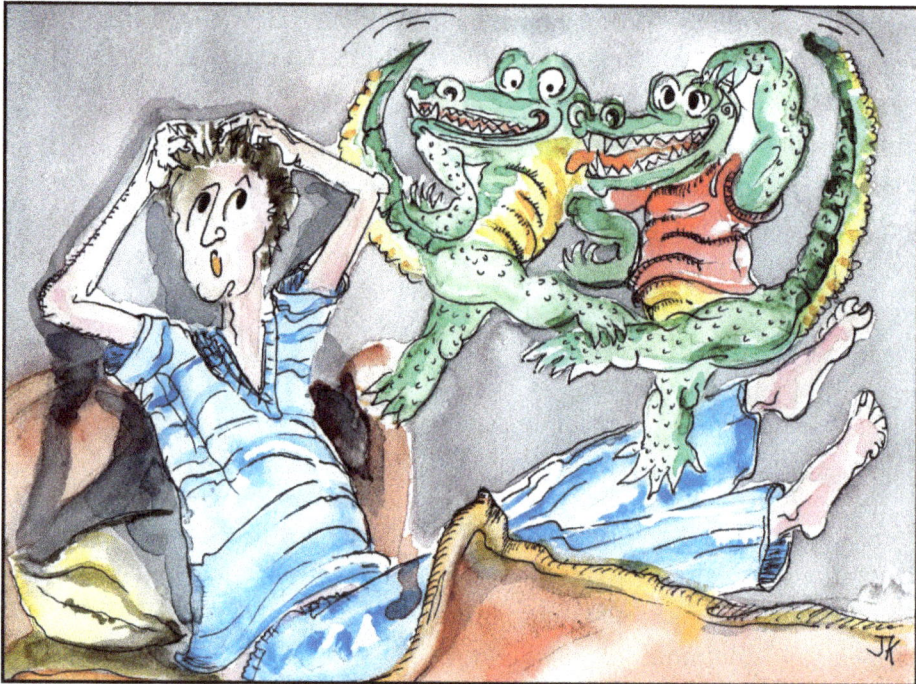

Will you please back off? I have enough alligators to deal with.

Testing in any form is not appropriate here. You have learned by this time that direct testing ("Do you remember?") is both unfair and demeaning to your friend. Indirect testing (for example, showing pictures of familiar people and places without asking for a response) can be just as bad. Your friend, despite their limitations, is still a sophisticated adult, who knows when you present the pictures, there is an implied association that you are looking for them to remember. There is no such thing as "no pressure" in this type of situation. You have inadvertently set them up to fail and this is very humiliating.

As caregivers, we all hope deep in our hearts that at points in time during the course of the disease our friend will reach back into Earth-reality, recognize us, and connect with our shared life experiences. Because of this hope, we are always listening, always hoping that the dreams on Altair will have components that *we* can relate to. Our mind is tuned to listen in this way, to reach out for lost connections. Can you see now that this is really just another form of testing? It is a bit like asking your teenage son questions about his evening out—where did you go, who was with you, what did you do? Really what you are doing is filtering your listening to watch for things you are concerned about, not truly listening to him.

With Alzheimer's disease, you know that the familiar landmarks you might find in one of these dreams (*today I am with Dad at work*) are false prophets tied to the bad Alzheimer's seed in your friend's mind, not the reality you share and understand here. And your joy and reinforcement of these memories, as if for a moment a door opened back into Earth-reality, is really based on an illusion.

Remember to simply join your partner's flow and relax. There is no need for you to solve anything (although assistance with the practical demands of daily routines is certainly needed). The world is not about your energy or your partner's. God is present here for both of you and supports your intentions even when they are masked by the noise of Altzair's dreams. The wisdom of the universe is yours for the asking.

* * *

More often than not, individuals and families struggling with Alzheimer's are struggling simultaneously with multiple other issues: their health, financial problems, logistic problems in caring for their loved one, stress, time away from other commitments, and many others. There is no simple fix for most, or perhaps, any of these issues, any more than there is a fix for the inevitability of death. But, there is help. It may be spiritual help, which never tires or fails and can take away the noise in your mind as you strive for solutions to problems that cannot be "solved" in any traditional sense. It may be help from organizations or individuals familiar with your situation.

Part of our expectation in Earth-time is that we can fix everything, that life is full of cause-effect events, and that when we do the right thing, a little flashing light appears showing PROBLEM SOLVED over and over in multiple colors. Alas, much of life and certainly everything to do with Alzheimer's is about a process, not a solution. And, as you know, a process can go on and on, much like a journey, and be filled with many detours and challenges, long before it reaches resolution. Take it a step at a time, a long moment at a time. Make decisions that protect you as a caregiver first, even if this runs counter to your thinking or our culture's thinking about how we care for the sick. Let me speak to you directly here. I forgive you, your partner with Alzheimer's forgives you, your family and friends forgive you, in advance, for all of the decisions you will need to make that have complex and temporary outcomes, not the hard and fast solutions that you would prefer. Take care of yourself and make decisions that respect your need for care!

HEAR MY VOICE

On Life Support

Please remember our agreements. I can speak to you today with the Comfort Card and hope that you can hear. While grateful for my physical wellness, day after day I live in agony and confusion over my mental deterioration. There are no long moments left for me and it also seems no relief.

A kinder God would have made a hospice for those suffering with Alzheimer's, but it doesn't exist. I long to be comfortable, but my mind rages with the frustration and confusion of living and not living. Is there no peace except in death?

The deep part of me that is still aware knows that this life is not sustainable for me, for you, for our family. I am caught in the limbo of Alzheimer's life support, sleeping, breathing, eating, but no longer living. How much longer must I go on like this? You are at your limits caring for me. I know you love me. Can you find a way to set me free?

I know that much of our life savings has been spent by you to care for me. We agreed that this would not be so. I know it makes you feel good to see me clean and cared for in this beautiful facility but I am beyond knowing or caring.

It is my time to go. Please do nothing to prolong my life. You cannot tell but my heart knows how you have sacrificed for me. You cannot tell but I love you so much. Please let me go.

Remember what we agreed? Every day from now on you will show me the Heaven Card, a wonderful card, that reminds me that I am in the last stages of hospice and it is time to die, peacefully, on my own. My mind and heart will understand and speed this process to bring me peace. That is my deepest wish.

I will see you again in the good times ...

Your loving mother,

Emilou

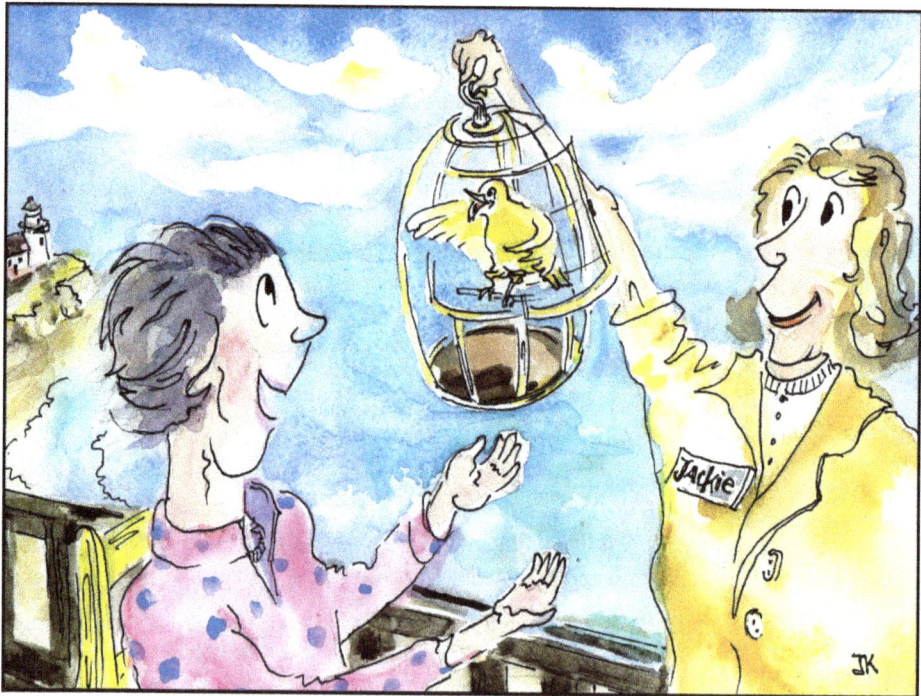

Nurse Jackie gives Katherine Emilou's surprise.

Chapter 10: Katherine and Emilou

Emilou: "I am dreaming all of the time now and you are in many of my dreams. In these dreams you are my child, my friend, my parent, and my guardian. I know that many times I can no longer express the joy that I feel when you are present, but you are patient with me, so patient, watching and hoping for a door to open that will connect us and trying not to show concern when it does not. I know you are here for me. My mind simply doesn't have the capability now to express my awareness of our connection directly.

"But you must know ... Every time we share a memory together that is good it becomes part of my dream. I am filled with joy on the inside and the outside. Being with you, listening to you, being touched by you brings many such memories into awareness.

"I can see it in your eyes. You think that I am not having a good day because I don't recognize you and because the connections that you offer to bring me temporarily into your Earth-time are not working. Yes, today is all about the Alzheimer's seed and my dreams—dreams that are not connected with our shared memories but only with Altzair. But this is neither good nor bad. It is just the way things are now. There is nothing wrong with me because I am not connecting with you in Earth-time. I am not having a bad day. Your presence and love and touch still warm my heart.

"I love you. I love your patience with me. It is tiring I know dealing with a helpless fool who cannot recognize you, respond to you appropriately, and needs assistance to dress, to eat, to bathe, to keep from messing things up. Do you see this smile on my face? Yes, it's the smile of a fool, but, it belongs to you."

Katherine: "I love you Mom. I'll miss you so much when you are gone."

Emilou: "Gone? I'm not going anywhere. You sound like I am going to die. I may be a fool, but I'm still young, in the prime of my life. In my dreams you are still a child. I have no fear of death. How did I get such an old body though? I'm confused."

Katherine: "I've watched you Mom, step by step, leave our shared world and step into your world of dreams. If you have found the Fountain of Youth, I am happy for you. Yes, I know that I am guilty of looking for the "good days" when you seem to recognize me or remember our connections from the past. But, I've been learning too. The joy of bringing you outside into the sun and wind to watch you smile with delight, or feeling you relax and take comfort in my touch as I sit with you and hold your hand, or just sitting quietly in your room listening to music—these are also good days."

Often after visiting Mom at lunchtime I would notice the treatment staff trying to calm Mary, a resident, who lived in Mom's wing. Mary would connect lunch and the early afternoon with picking up her daughter Jill from school and would become very upset when she was told not to leave the facility to get her. Then, suddenly, after a month of this behavior, it stopped. I asked the nurse about it and she explained, our Alzheimer's expert, Jytte, happened to be here last week and noticed Mary was upset, so she simply reminded her that she had previously made arrangements with a friend to pick up Jill. Now we all use this approach whenever Mary has a problem.

Emilou: "My world is connected to yours by hundreds of tiny luminous strands, fragile but as strong as a spider's web. Can you see them? At times they are so real that when you prompt me I can grab one and almost travel back into your world, for just a moment, to be with you. Every strand carries the precious seed of a long moment, waiting to happen. Each day though, a few more disappear. Soon there will be nothing left to tether my planet to yours. But this doesn't matter. Your presence is a part of me in so many other ways, and as long as I am dreaming, your touch, your warmth, your smile will be part of the dream, bringing hope and richness and familiarity."

Katherine: "Please don't go Mom. I see no strands but those that connect you to my world, our world at one time, a connection that grows weaker and weaker."

Emilou: "Don't worry. When all of these tiny strands are gone, I will still be fine. Please do not be afraid for me. It is you I am concerned about. When there are no more 'good days' for me in your world, how will you deal with this? You will think of me as gone, when really I am not. I will still be here, living with the seed of Altzair in my mind. When you look for me in your heart, I will be there. I will always be there."

116

Katherine: "Mom, I am afraid. I don't know what to do. I don't want to lose you but I cannot stop what is happening to you. I remember your dad, Fodda, and the years that he lived disconnected from all of us. I'm your daughter. I want to be with you and bring you comfort and love as you have done so many years for me. I don't want to lose you."

Emilou: "I have my own journey to make now. To you, it will seem as though I have simply gone away and am dead to your world, but that is not the case. In my dreams on Altzair, I am very much alive and very much open to you through all of the other channels of communication that you have learned in this book. Your visits will still be important to me but it is OK to begin to turn loose and come less frequently. You have been here for me for many years and it is time to begin to live more now in your world, with Denise and your family.

"This may sound cruel but I will not notice. Soon the dream will be all consuming and there will be no strands left for me to travel that connect us in a shared reality.

"I have something for you."

The nursing home has a locked Alzheimer's unit where residents live who might tend to wander or harm themselves. Not all residents in this wing are in wheelchairs thus the need to have locked doors.

One evening after dinner I was sitting with my mom quietly watching TV when the door to the locked unit opened and an aide was escorting two gentlemen from the locked area. As they approached a small conference room, one of the patients turned to me and said, "We are having a board meeting, will be discussing business, and then off for a boy's night out." As I watched the aide seat the men at the conference table, she handed them newspapers, pens, pencils, and then closed the door. What a great plan to acknowledge that these men had been productive businessmen and although Alzheimer's has taken that ability away ... the men didn't know it. They were being treated with respect for who they were, not what they had become.

Katherine and Emilou have been sitting outside in the sun watching the cumulus clouds build over the Atlantic Ocean. Jackie, Emilou's favorite nurse, approaches and hands Katherine a small cage. Inside is a green parakeet.

Jackie sees Katherine's puzzled look, smiles, and gently touches her shoulder.

"Do you remember Billy?"

"Of course, I brought him to Mom. She talked about a parakeet for weeks, then seemed to be happy when I surprised her with him. Why is he here now?"

"Actually, I think Emilou wants you to take him home."

Katherine looks at Emilou, who is smiling as she watches Billy move around the cage, then suddenly is distracted and looks away.

Emilou: *"Yes, please take Billy with you. He has been waiting, you see, a long time to go home with you."*

Katherine, smiling now, gives Emilou a suspicious look.

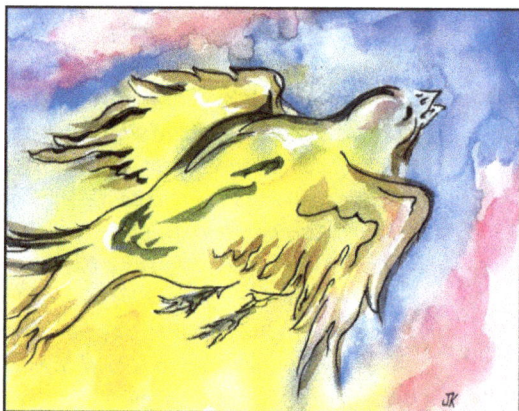

I have a present for you Katherine.

"A parakeet, Mom? You want me to take Billy home? Why?"

Emilou looks briefly at Katherine, at Billy, and then looks back at the clouds, nodding her head and remaining silent.

Emilou: *"It's time Katherine. Soon all my connections to our shared world will be gone. Billy, however, lives in both realms. He has been with me on Altair and also in your world. He lives now with a part of me inside him that will be there forever. Please take him with you to remind you that while I cannot show it, I will always be part of you and part of your world even though it will appear that I have gone.*

"I have very few long moments left for you in this world, but every time you see Billy you will be reminded of one of those moments that we have already shared. Remember the trip to Chattanooga when Richard got into so much trouble and how you laughed and laughed until you discovered that it was your sheets that he had put into the bathtub!

"Billy, you see, is my tether. He will connect us now and so instead of waiting and hoping that I will join you for a long moment he will remind you

that the moment already exists in your mind, that you can remember me, remember us, in our shared world filled with memories anytime you choose.

"I love you so much. Thank you for caring for me. Please care for yourself now."

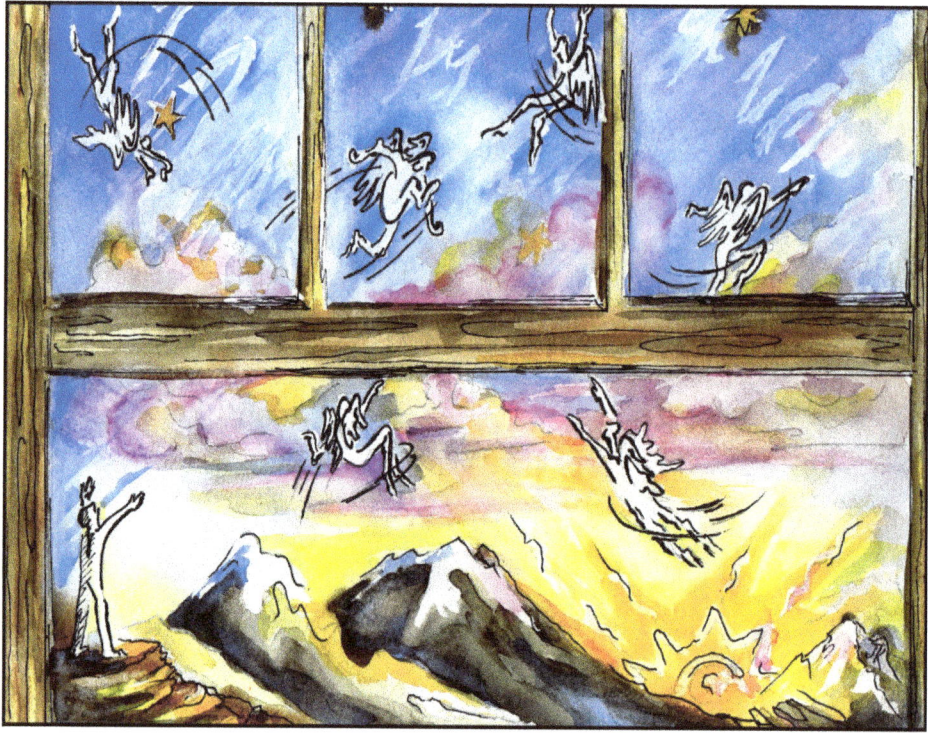

Opening the window to the universe

Chapter 11: The Doors of Birth and Death

We take the concept of our shared, consensual reality so much for granted that it is essentially invisible to us. The colors we see; the shapes of things; our sense of taste and smell; how you are expected to behave in a variety of social settings; the rules for driving a car, dining in a restaurant, playing baseball; facial expressions; physical responses such as holding, caressing, or hitting; the meaning of familiar phrases and words in conversations; the significance of key agreements or contracts such as a marriage or a loan for a car; and thousands of others.

The connections between the billions of neurons in your brain and most every experience in the world are complex learned associations reinforced and shaped over time through our agreements to share the same reality.

You were not always constructed this way. At birth, some of these terns such as the perception of faces or expressions appear to be hardwired, but most everything else, from how to use your hands and arms to toss a ball or eat to understanding what things in the world are safe or dangerous, need to be learned. Social agreements tend to be family-oriented and limited until you start school and then they develop rapidly on many dimensions. There is a son why imaginary playmates tend to disappear in kindergarten or the first grade. Children quickly learn that experiences that cannot be shared and consensually validated are not "real" in most cultures and therefore not reinforced, and this pattern continues on throughout our lives.

Alzheimer's disease, of course, disrupts these patterns in a very destructive manner because the model of the world that we carry in our minds is especially vulnerable to corruption in the areas that underlie our shared agreements about reality. As you know, touch, taste, color, or music, many skills, life experiences, or even some simple social agreements, such as how to greet a friend, are likely to be less affected. What hurts the most is that the Alzheimer's seed, once planted in the mind, quickly begins to destroy the anchors that tie the mind to our shared, consensual reality so our model of the world is no longer valid, and, like a poorly constructed robot, it no longer understands the rules that it was carefully programmed to operate by because it cannot separate what is real from what is not.

When we view Alzheimer's from the beginning and end of life, however, our perspective can change and the hard-fought battles to maintain the dance of real/not real or Earth-time/Altzair-time become irrelevant. At the edges of birth and death, the boundaries that we construct and maintain all of our lives between ourselves as separate individuals and ourselves as separate unique beings who are somehow different from and not connected to the rest of the universe disappear. Look into the eyes of any infant and you will not only see the innocence that comes from the absence of any social programming, a blank slate of sorts, you will also see a window that ties back genetically to thousands of prior generations, to the wisdom of the Earth and all things that exist on the Earth, and to the spiritual dimensions that we all seek but often block with our religions and social conventions.

Death is much more about the living than the dead. I've never been particularly concerned about my own death, but from the moment my son Logan was born, I was very concerned about his death and wanted to do everything possible to be sure he was safe and protected. His early death changed my own life in ways that I could never imagine. Unconsciously, for many years, I blocked the grace of being loved and comforted by others fearing, in my commitment to them, I would suffer another loss.

The same window opens again as we approach death. It is the gateway to all things shared, open, and connected in the universe. In the end, there are no boundaries. We are all one grand being connected not only to our past but to the history of all things on the Earth. The next time a friend or family member approaches death, look through the pain and discomfort (if this is present) and into what is behind the eyes, and you will be seeing the same unbounded universe that is present at birth. The march to death for a family dealing with Alzheimer's can be stressful to the point of being tragic on many dimensions (if this is the choice that is made). In the end, however, the Alzheimer's seed cannot take away the connections between the mind and the universe of all minds. Just as a friendly touch, a smile, or a walk in the sun almost always connects with an Alzheimer's patient, at death, the universe of peace and calm is waiting to embrace another soul in a time and place where our artificial, shared models of reality no longer matter.

Birth and death, with life on Earth or Altzair in between, take us into and out of a shared, consensual reality. Living any life advances us steadily in a march back to the planet of our birth. In the beginning it was filled with the wisdom of genetic history, a vast template going back to the beginning of life on Earth. In the end it is rich with the lakes and forests of our memories, layer after layer deposited for many years, waiting to be shared with future generations.

Remember when you were younger, and as you looked back on the previous year, you could see how much you and the world had changed? Then gradually, as you aged, the years became more similar and the differences less pronounced. Alzheimer's sends this natural process into a repetitive loop much like the loop on a damaged CD that plays the same notes over and over. When you are in the loop, there is no place to stand to look back and view last year or this year or yesterday. There is only a distorted scratchy version of "now," which can be momentarily normal, but is more likely to be filled with uncertainty and confusion.

As the end approaches in Earth-reality you seem to be helpless. Your caregivers watch you as your physical and mental health continue to deteriorate, day by day. What they don't understand is that on Altzair these struggles don't exist. Here you are fearless because the concept of death and dying no longer exists. Here you are ageless because, long ago, your mind retreated into the past when you were young and healthy and filled with love and energy and thousands of luminous bands connected you with every dimension of the universe. Here, in the deepest parts of your consciousness, you are experiencing the Fountain of Youth because the recent memories, the shell of you as a person with Alzheimer's disease, no longer prevail.

Yes, part of you may long for a transition to death filled with a full spectrum of life's memories from childhood to old age. It is not to be. Your march on Altzair will be to a different drummer as you cross over, bringing none of the excess baggage from these last years, none of the confusion, conflict, and pain, only the essence of who you are and what you became in the heart of your life. In your eyes I see joy not fear or conflict or confusion. Given a choice, you would not have chosen a path through Altzair. Having no choice, you embrace these last moments of eternal youth in our shared world and move on with no regrets.

* * *

Emilou: "My days are like that now. In the beginning my dreams were wanderings in the vast landscape of past experiences.   I roamed from one end of Altzair to the other, capturing moments that blended with my memories of you and your visits and of your love. Now my dreams are a wasteland of dreams of dreams of dreams.   Night and day are all the same now, an ongoing dream that

never seems to end. Imagine entering a movie theater and never leaving. I long for an intermission. There are no long moments. There is quiet but not stillness. My dreams are like watching ten movies with the scenes broken apart arbitrarily and then stitched randomly together.

Although I have no evidence that Emilou has actually seen a "red-headed" angel, it has appeared several times in my life.

On the night before his death, my son Logan sat with me on the top of a mountain where we were camping. We had spent the day with a friend rock climbing. He described his plans for his life, his love of music, his concerns for his mom starting a new career, and finally, the visits from the angel. The angel, I questioned? Yes, a red-haired angel had visited with him several times in the past month. The purpose of the visits was not clear but he sensed both the power and love coming from the angel and was comforted by her presence. Less than twenty-four hours later, he would be in my arms, unconscious and badly injured from a fall, his last breaths as faint as a dying ember, delivered to heaven I am sure by that same angel.

"But I can feel a change coming. It started about a month ago with the red-headed angel. She was in one of my dreams, and when she touched me, the dream was whole and clear and filled with places and people I had never seen before. But I wasn't afraid. It was very peaceful. Now she is with me almost every day. The last time she visited, when she left, she walked through a door that remained partially open. The light is so bright I cannot see beyond it.

"She tried to explain that soon I would be dreaming a new dream, the 'dream of life,' and that all of the old dreams would disappear. She said that you will not be in the new dream, nor will any of my family, but that I would not be afraid. You will always be with me, she said, but the dream belongs to my future not my past.

"I love you. Goodbye."

* * *

I hope that this book has given you some insight into the deep well of Alzheimer's disease that we are just beginning to fathom. While imagining this conversation with Emilou that is peaceful and spiritual (and I wish that for you), it cannot be denied that life is often more complicated than that. You know of course, by now, that you cannot substantially alter the path that your friend with Alzheimer's is on, because like all life, it is a march to death. What you can do is alter your life so that you are more at peace and less in the mode of "fixing things." You can accept and understand and listen more and open the many channels of communication described in this book. Despite the decline of your friend on so many levels, their essence remains intact. Your gift to them will be in seeing their essence and reflecting it back to them with love, unconditional acceptance, and respect. When the time comes and they pass on, the gift you will receive will be the knowledge that you were there for them with the blessing of many long moments.

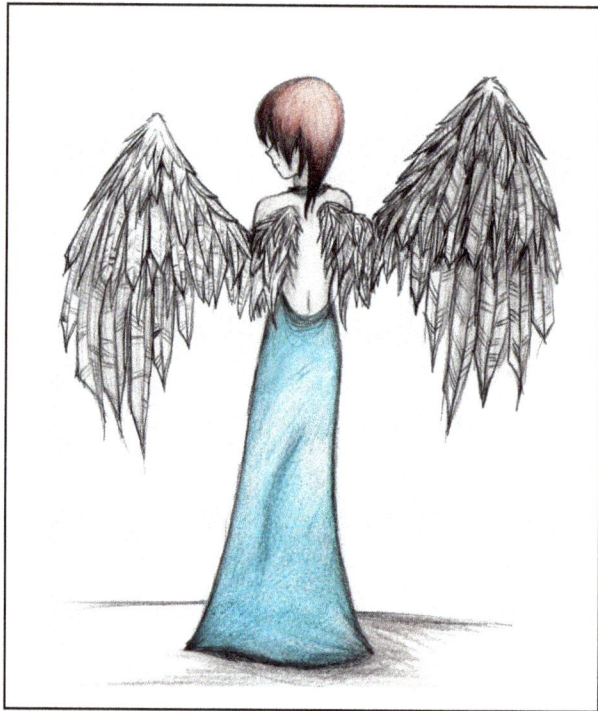

The red-haired angel

Chapter 12: Closure

Emilou: "It is very cold on my planet today. Even the pleasant memories of you and Tim and Mom, as we were in the 1950s, can no longer warm me. I think of you, my dear child, with love, but those moments are fleeting, offering only a quick glimpse into the past, then shattering like broken glass, with a thousand fragmented thoughts pulling in many directions.

"Night and day on Altzair are all the same now, an ongoing dream that never seems to end. I am always trapped in a dark tunnel. I long for the steps leading back to the sunlight.

"The candle of eternal youth is tempting, but not in this lonely shell, helpless, weak, aged, and disconnected from so many things on Earth that I remember and long for.

"Lately I have been seeing the door left slightly ajar by the angel in many of my dreams. It is a door with people behind it. I think I see Mom and my children, Gail and James, there, waiting, but I am not sure. When I turn toward it, the light from the sun is so bright they disappear. Gail was speaking to me but I could not hear."

* * *

"This morning, finally, a change. I am very happy.

"Gail came through the door. I could see the light as before, then, a shadow and suddenly Gail was next to me. She is so beautiful."

* * *

"I am ready.

"Gail tells me that today will be a day of transition. She has combed my hair. I am wearing the black dress Mom gave me for Christmas. She is so beautiful.

"She has explained that neither the Earth nor Altzair are real but just convenient constructions of my mind, but today I will experience the reality that all living things share with no artificial layers of language or human constructs.

"We sit quietly, waiting, her hand on my arm.

"'I am ready,' I say, watching the open door.

"Did it just come closer?"

* * *

As I write these closing words in the spring of 2013, I can report that Emilou has made it through another year, which, with failing physical health, and celebrating her hundredth birthday, is quite an accomplishment! During Katherine's visits, she spent much of her time on Altzair, living as a child or young adult and struggling to connect these memories with the present. Katherine today is a familiar friend who visits often but not the daughter Katherine that Emilou remembers. Of course, on Altzair, these past connections have little meaning in the present, at least to Emilou.

I know in my heart that she is ready and that soon, this year perhaps, God will grant her wish and she, Gail, James, and many others from her life will be reunited.

Emilou has been fortunate to be near family and to have a generous, kind caregiver such as Katherine present, but her physical health and longevity, just as with her father, have added years of stress, uncertainty, and some financial hardship for the family as retirement accounts, intended to last many more years, were quickly consumed with the intensive care required.

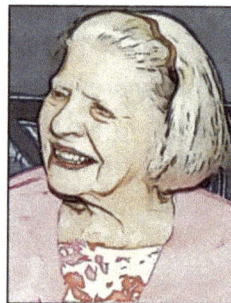

Emilou at 100

Unlike most native cultures on the planet, our culture fears death and places an artificial value on "living" long past the point when life, by any standard but biological, is meaningful. The concept of euthanasia, even when the mind is completely healthy, is so contrary to our cultural norms that we make it inaccessible to those in need and punish those who have the courage and grace to assist them. Could there be such a thing for late stage Alzheimer's patients? Probably not, because most with late stage Alzheimer's are not capable of making a clear rational decision regarding ending their life. Or at least this is what we hold to be true in our culture. But what is the alternative? Continuing a life that in many cases no longer has meaning and is filled with frustration and suffering.

I wish for many things for those touched by Alzheimer's, but my greatest wish and the focus of this book has to do with having options. We, as a busy, verbally oriented culture, have options to open meaningful channels of communication that endure throughout the course of the disease. We have the option to broaden our understanding of human consciousness to include non-verbal forms of communication, and finally to change our perception of Alzheimer's from that of a death march (which of course applies to all of us) to that of a meaningful but handicapped style of living from the moment of the diagnosis to the end.

We don't abandon our loved ones with terminal cancer or other diseases despite the inevitability of the final outcome. We give them hope. We nourish them. We change our perception of life to embrace them and their needs.

This is also possible with your friend or spouse with Alzheimer's disease. The first step, however, is a big one, because it involves expanding your perception of reality. As a caregiver, I invite you to broaden your view of logical, consensually shared reality to include images, emotions, feelings, and dreams. With this expanded view, there is more room for diversity and more options for communication. The door is open for all of us.

I have had the privilege of assisting family and friends many times when a loved one was near death. I try to help the individual who is dying embrace death graciously and without fear by letting go (often this is easy because most people at this stage are ready) and then I tackle the real problem: helping the family "let go" so that their energy is not focused on extending the life of their loved one but on intentionally "saying goodbye" so that the individual is not fighting to stay alive for the family's sake.

This simple idea of giving a dying person permission to die is very important and yet, outside of hospice, as a culture we fight this idea so fiercely that many individuals, on their deathbed, feel guilty about passing, as if this most natural of processes is letting their family down. With Alzheimer's patients, as with anyone with a terminal illness, I encourage you to talk about death in a gentle, loving way. While the waking conscious mind may not understand, there are other layers of consciousness that will hear your words and are craving the blessing of ending a life that no longer makes sense.

On my last visit, I spent fifteen minutes alone with Emilou, talking about the beauty, serenity, and closure that was waiting for her in death, when she was ready.

Appendices

Appendix A: The Alzheimer's Cards

What are they?
The Alzheimer's Card Decks are sets of cards designed to be used as a communication device during the middle and late stages of Alzheimer's disease when verbal/logical speech patterns have deteriorated. The cards are intended, largely for the Alzheimer's patient, to provide a voice expressing their needs, feelings, and intentions. Many of the cards can also be used by caregivers to communicate especially when a normal conversation is not possible. Caregivers of course have needs and feelings and many times would like to share a message with their companion but cannot.

How will I use them?
As Alzheimer's disease progresses, many of the normal channels of communication with your friends such as having a conversation or writing a letter will diminish over time until they no longer become a reliable way of sharing your feelings, ideas, or needs. As you can already imagine, this deterioration in everyday communication ability is enormously frustrating especially when you want or need to share what is on your mind with caregivers but cannot. The Alzheimer's Cards offer a new way of communicating that will remain alive and working long after traditional speech becomes problematic. At any time you choose, you can use the cards to express a feeling, an idea, or a need simply by going to the deck, extracting a card or cards, and sharing them. It is that simple.

Why will it work?
The cards work because, while your mind will lose its ability to hang onto the kinds of details and logic that we commonly use when we talk, it will retain many of the core images and ideas contained in the card for much longer. For example, the details about a specific event in your life involving a parent may be lost or, if available, difficult to connect in any way to your current experiences and conversations. However, the idea of a parent and the feelings that parent brings to mind—perhaps love or strength or protection—are still accessible to you and will be for some time. Viewing the Parent Card can help to evoke these feelings in your own mind or, by giving the card to a caregiver, allow you to share this feeling with others. When you can no longer communicate easily with words, the simple act of sharing a card can be priceless.

The two types of Alzheimer's Cards

Alzheimer's Cards are divided into two groups, the Early Stage Cards for individuals in the beginning or middle stages and the Late Stage Cards for individuals with significant communication problems common to the later stages of the disease process. As described above, the greatest need is probably for the Late Stage Cards since communication in the late stages is challenging and the available resources to help quite limited. Late Stage Cards are simpler, focused on immediate needs and emotions, and if imagery is present, it is very clear and linked to the message on the card.

Is there a protocol for using the cards?

There are many options for using the Early Stage Cards including some standard layouts or patterns described in the instruction booklet. Because the standard deck of Late Stage Cards represents a tool deliberately designed to help the Alzheimer's patient with basic communication, I do recommend following a well-defined protocol that is practiced in the early/middle stages so that its use in the late stages will be familiar. The process begins with a favorite piece of music used to signal that the next few minutes are about communication. After approximately one minute, the deck of cards is put on the table with the COMMUNICATE or I HAVE SOMETHING TO SAY Card arranged on top. Once this card is selected, the process can begin. Please see the Alzheimer's Cards booklet for more information on the next steps in using the cards in both early/middle and late stages.

Where can I find a deck of cards to use?

You may already know the answer to this question since many copies of *The Long Moment* come with a set of Alzheimer's Cards included and a book of instructions on using the cards. If you purchased the book without cards, please go to the website AlzheimersCards.com and you can find a number of options for ordering Early or Late Stage Decks or making your own deck of cards. You can also download the instruction booklet for using the cards.

Special Agreements

The next few pages contain several proposed agreements intended to help with long-term planning for family and caregivers. Please realize that these are simply draft agreements designed to create options for individuals with Alzheimer's disease and their caregivers similar to the options available for other diseases. None of these suggested agreements have any legal standing! Please use them as templates to create your own agreements or just to support conversations on these important topics.

Appendix B: My Alzheimer's Choice Book

Recognizing that my diagnosis of Alzheimer's disease will bring about a steady deterioration of my mental and physical abilities over time such that at some point I will no longer be able to take an active part in decisions about my care or my future, I choose to let this booklet stand as an expression of my choices, wishes, and directions while I am still healthy and of sound mind.

In loving appreciation for my current and future friends, family, and other care-givers who graciously and courageously share the burden of this disease with me.

Signed_____

Witness_____

Witness_____

Date_____

Choices in the Early Stages While I Am Still Mentally Able to Share the Same Reality with You Most of the Time

1. Where I want to live.

_____

2. Things that are important to me in the environment where I am living.

_____

3. How I want to spend my time.

_____

4. Who I want to see during the early stages of the disease.

_____

5. How much attention I need from family and friends.

_____

6. What things I want you to avoid doing.

_____

7. How I want you to respond to my frustration as my abilities to cope in our shared reality are diminished.

_____

8. How I want you to show love and caring for me.

_____

9. How I intend to show my love and consideration for you.

_____

10. How I want you to care for yourself. Here are some boundaries.

_____

Choices in the Middle Stages When My Reality and Yours Begin to Differ Much of the Time

1. Where I want to live.

_____

2. Things that are important to me in the environment where I am living.

_____

3. How I want to spend my time.

_____

4. Who I want to see during the middle stages of the disease.

_____

5. How much attention I need from family and friends.

_____

6. What things I want you to avoid doing.

_____

7. How I want you to respond to my frustration as my abilities to cope in our shared reality are diminished.

_____

8. How I want you to show love and caring for me.

_____

9. How I intend to show my love and consideration for you.

_____

10. How I want you to care for yourself. Here are some boundaries.

_____

Choices in the Late Stages When I Am No Longer Living in Your World

1. Where I want to live.

_____

2. Things that are important to me in the environment where I am living.

_____

3. How I want to spend my time.

_____

4. Who I want to see during the late stages of the disease.

_____

5. How much attention I need from family and friends.

_____

6. What things I want you to avoid doing.

_____

7. How I want you to respond to my frustration as my abilities to cope in our shared reality are diminished.

_____

8. How I want you to show love and caring for me.

_____

9. How I intend to show my love and consideration for you.

_____

10. How I want you to care for yourself. Here are some boundaries.

_____

Appendix C: How I Want to Be Remembered

I recognize that in the middle and late stages of Alzheimer's I will most likely be a stranger to you handicapped in many ways that make a natural, social transition from life to death unlikely. I *do not* wish to be remembered as this stranger whom you will recognize but no longer know. Please remember me through the window of our history together when I was healthy and shared the same world with you. I know that I will grieve the loss of this world as darkness descends on Altzair but will be helpless to do anything about it. You, on the other hand, can bring me love, and hope, and courage by remembering who I really am and finding ways to share this with me when you visit. Even though I may be a stranger to you and not responsive, please remind me who I am with words, with touch, with any personal Alzheimer's Cards we have created, with visits outside to places that you know I love, and with any other action I will appreciate. Part of me will know. Part of me resonates inside with the sound of joy as you help me remember *me* without testing. In my passing, it is these moments I will take with me on the way to heaven.

Here is how I would like you to remember me:

_____

_____

_____

_____

_____

_____

_____

_____

(Signed and Dated)

Appendix D: Alzheimer's Hospice Agreement

1. PARTIES TO THE AGREEMENT

This is an Agreement between _____ (PATIENT) and my family, friends, or other caregivers represented by the following person or persons:

_____
_____(CAREGIVERS).

2. NOT A LEGAL HOSPICE AGREEMENT

All Parties to the Agreement understand that this is not a legally binding Hospice Agreement but rather a special agreement intended to offer the grace, clarity, and intent of hospice care to late stage Alzheimer's patients where the guidelines associated with a traditional understanding of hospice may not apply. The existence of this Agreement is in no way intended to substitute for or replace a more formal, legally binding Hospice Agreement that provides basic services and other benefits to an individual in the last stages of their life.

3. SPECIAL DEFINITION OF SUFFERING FOR ALZHEIMER'S PATIENTS

This Agreement acknowledges that most individuals with Alzheimer's disease experience a diminished quality of life in the late stages of the disease that, if given a choice, would under normal circumstances lead them to not extend this life. However, because the conditions and symptoms of the Alzheimer's patient often fall outside the boundaries of traditional Hospice Agreements or Living Wills, the ongoing mental suffering and anguish of the disease, which has no current treatment, is maintained indefinitely as long as the body is physically healthy.

4. DECISION TO EXTEND THE DEFINITON OF HOSPICE TO INLCUDE MY MENTAL SUFFERING

In signing this Agreement as a healthy individual experiencing the symptoms of early stage Alzheimer's disease and being of sound mind, I wish to make it clear to my CAREGIVERS that I choose NOT TO PROLONG MY SUFFERING IN THE LATE STAGES OF THE DISEASE PROCESS WHEN MY MIND IS NO LONGER PART OF OUR SHARED WORLD. Indications that I have reached this point in the progression of the disease include the following:

- I do not remember you, my CAREGIVERS, and our shared experiences together.
- I have lost all sense of the past and the future and am living in brief moments that recycle over and over during your visits.
- There are few or no things that bring me joy during the day. I am physically alive but mentally not connected to the world.
- I have lost my ability to communicate with you.
- It takes a full-time person or staff to sustain me and care for me during the normal daily routines of waking, bathing, dressing, using the toilet, dining, and other behaviors.

5. UNDERSTANDING THE SPIRIT OF HOSPICE IN MY CIRCUMSTANCES

I understand that hospice care, in general, is palliative not curative in nature and is designed to provide for the relief of my symptoms such as pain and physical discomfort as well as to support my emotional and spiritual needs. With this Agreement I am asking for an expansion of the definition of hospice to include my mental suffering that is an inevitable part of Alzheimer's disease. In making this statement, I also understand that unlike most individuals in hospice, I will not have a choice to change or withdraw from this Agreement because by the time it is relevant I will no longer understand it.

6. DECISION NOT TO EXTEND MY LIFE

My Living Will describes the conditions under which I wish to have or not have special treatments or procedures, such as resuscitation, performed to extend my life. In signing this Agreement, I am saying that during the later stages of Alzheimer's disease, when the conditions described in #4 exist for me, if there is a process occurring that can end my life in a comfortable, natural way, I choose to allow this to happen. I understand that this is a CHOICE between being physically alive but not really part of the world and suffering, every day, from the mental disruption created by the disease, and leaving this world through death by natural processes. I choose to die rather than have you extend my life. I also request that you prepare me for this death by reminding me during your visits, when we reach this critical period, that I have your permission to leave, so that the part of my mind that will understand you and may be holding onto life because of you can let go.

Thank you in advance for your love and consideration in honoring this Agreement.

Name and Signature of Patient:

_____

Name and Signature of Caregiver(s):

_____

Acknowledgments

Any book project, large or small, requires lots of help and support and patience from those who work with the author. I am most grateful to the following individuals:

Laurel Ornitz, my editor, who turned my rough manuscript into a book and always had the right "push" when needed to bring this project to closure.

Carolyn Moore and Jytte Lokvig, my Alzheimer's experts, who coached me through the different sections of the book with their expertise on Alzheimer's disease, their stories and examples that grounded my writing in many places, and their patience with my naiveté.

Glenys Carl, author and founder of Coming Home Connection, for her wisdom and support on many dimensions to see this project finished.

Jean Kithil, the talented artist who provided most of the beautiful color illustrations in the book and Cindy Lux who designed the cover.

George Burdeau, friend and screenwriter, who pushed me to make the book more personal and less abstract.

My wife Marilyn, who supported my work in many ways and with her own time helped to free my time to write and create.

Vadim Kovalenko, my friend and programmer from Minsk, who constructed the technology and web tools for the TheAlzheimersCards.com website. His work is the reason they will be widely available.

Finally, and obviously not least, my heart goes out to the book's real heroes, Katherine and Emilou (and my other family members), who not only allowed me to write a book about them, sharing their personal history, but in Katherine's case, helped with many of the true stories that you see in boxes throughout the book.

I'm sure that Dad is a little surprised to see me write a book on Alzheimer's but smiling nonetheless.

About the Author

Dr. Richard Fenker is an Emeritus Professor of Psychology at TCU, inventor, writer, artist, and forecaster. He is the author of more than 500 published articles and technical briefs, a dozen books, and many papers on astronomy, mathematical psychology, pattern recognition, cognitive psychology, learning, environmental design, consciousness, sport psychology, forecasting and retail location analysis. Many of his books, on learning (*Stop Studying Start Learning: How to Jumpstart Your Brain*), photography (*Where Rainbows Wait for Rain: The Big Bend Country*), and location forecasting (*The Site Book: A Guide to Commercial Real Estate Evaluation*) are still available on Amazon.

His interest in Alzheimer's disease stems from his experiences with family members and friends and his background in the study of human consciousness. His three books on learning all emphasize the importance of using left- and right-brain consciousness for studying. He has thought for many years that part of the isolation experienced by Alzheimer's patients comes from our general lack of understanding of the different layers of human consciousness and the role they play in communication.

Richard lives with his wife Marilyn in Santa Fe, New Mexico. You can visit his website at richardfenker.com.

www.ingramcontent.com/pod-product-compliance
Lightning Source LLC
Chambersburg PA
CBHW080044280326
41935CB00014B/1782